Gastric Carcinoma

Jürgen Hotz Hans-Joachim Meyer
H.-J. Schmoll
Editors

Gastric Carcinoma

Classification, Diagnosis, and Therapy

With 56 Figures, 14 in Full Color

Springer-Verlag
Berlin Heidelberg New York
London Paris Tokyo

Jürgen Hotz, M.D.
Professor of Medicine
Head, Department of Gastroenterology and Oncology
General Hospital
Celle, FRG

Hans-Joachim Meyer, M.D.
Professor of Surgery
Department of Surgery
Division of Abdominal and Transplantation Surgery
Medical University of Hannover
Hannover, FRG

H.-J. Schmoll, M.D.
Professor
Department of Hematology/Oncology
Medical University of Hannover
Hannover, FRG

The publication of this book was made possible by Merck Sharp & Dohme.

Translation of *Magenkarzinom*/Klassification, Diagnostik und stadiengerechte Therapie

Library of Congress Cataloging-in-Publication Data
Magenkarzinom. English
Gastric carcinoma : classification, diagnosis, and therapy / J. Hotz, H.-J. Meyer, H.-J. Schmoll, editors.
p. cm.
Translation of: Magenkarzinom.
Result of a workshop held in Neu-Isenburg, Germany, Oct. 30–31, 1987: sponsored by Frost Pharma.
ISBN-13:978-0-387-96955-8 (pbk. : U.S.) : $39.95 (est.)
1 Stomach–Cancer–Congresses. I. Hotz, J. II. Meyer, H.-J. (Hans-Joachim) III. Schmoll, H.-J. (Hans-Joachim) IV. Frost Pharma, V. Title.
[DNLM: 1. Stomach Neoplasms–congresses. WI 320 M192 1987a)
RC280.S8M24132 1989
616.99'433–dc20
DNLM/DLC
for Library of Congress 89-11277
CIP

Typeset by Publishers Service, Bozeman, Montana.

9 8 7 6 5 4 3 2 1

ISBN-13:978-0-387-96955-8 e-ISBN-13:978-1-4612-3636-8
DOI: 10.1007/978-1-4612-3636-8

Preface

In recent years the study of gastric carcinoma has been neglected by gastroenterology. This can be gleaned from the major topics featured at national and international gastroenterology conferences, which largely ignore the malignant diseases of the gastrointestinal tract, with the exception of carcinoma of the colon. A partial explanation may be that the endoscopic and histologic diagnosis of gastric carcinoma, including the detection of early cancer, has been honed, and it appears that little of new scientific value is expected to be gained therefrom. In many cases conservative therapeutic efforts involving patients who were inoperable or whose surgery was incurable have been frustrating, giving rise to a rather fatalistic attitude among gastroenterologists where this disease is concerned. In contrast, the topic "gastric carcinoma" continues to have a decisive influence on the interest of the discipline of general surgery in the search for an adequate surgical approach. Recently, oncology—often unobserved by gastroenterology—has made progress in this field and attained the first true chemotherapeutic successes. Thus, today there is no longer doubt that gastric cancer is sensitive, in a relative sense, to cytostatic drugs compared with other tumors of the gastrointestinal tract, eg, carcinomas of the colon, pancreas, and liver. Effective palliation in advanced stages as well as a combination of surgical and chemotherapeutic modalities of treatment lend hope for the future.

Therefore, we are of the opinion that it is time to unite the aforementioned disciplines—including pathology—in order to take stock of these new developments; the goal is to establish guidelines and advice for the treatment and guidance of patients with gastric cancer that will be valid for us today. The book at hand is the result of a workshop with this same goal. The individual contributions reproduced step-by-step the present level of knowledge in epidemiology, etiopathology, classification, and diagnosis as well as in surgical therapy and oncologic chemotherapeutic possibilities. Finally, we will present practical, current guidelines concerning the stage-specific diagnosis and therapy of gastric carcinoma, which were worked out in joint discussions, and which are oriented to the present level of knowledge and future prospects.

We would like to express our deep gratitude to the sponsor of this workshop, Frost Pharma, and to Merck Sharp & Dohme for its valuable support, as well as to Springer-Verlag, and to Mr. Lewerich and Mrs. Botsch in particular, for their dedicated collaboration in the production of this work.

J. Hotz, Celle, Federal Republic of Germany
H.-J. Meyer, Hannover, Federal Republic of Germany
H.-J. Schmoll, Hannover, Federal Republic of Germany

Contents

Part V. Summary

Contributors

W. Achterrath, M.D., Department of Surgery, University of Münster, 4400 Münster, FRG

K. Buhl, M.D., Department of Surgery, University of Heidelberg, Heidelberg, FRG

Howard Warren Bruckner, M.D., Associate Professor of Neoplastic Diseases and Medicine, Mount Sinai School of Medicine, New York, NY 10029, USA

Gernot Feifel, M.D., Professor of Surgery, Surgical University Clinic, 6650 Homburg/Saar, FRG

U. Fink, M.D., Department of Surgery, Division of Medical Oncology, University of Münster, 4400 Münster, FRG

H. Goebell, M.D., Professor, Section of Gastroenterology, Medical Clinic and Policlinic, 4300 Essen, FRG

Reinhard Grote, M.D., Department of Diagnostic Radiology, Medical University of Hannover, 3000 Hannover, FRG

G. Heidl, M.D., Surgical Clinic and Policlinic of the Westf. Wilhelms University, 4400 Münster, FRG

P. Heintz, M.D., Department of Diagnostic Radiology, Medical University of Hannover, 3000 Hannover, FRG

C. Herfarth, M.D., Professor, Surgical Clinic, University of Heidelberg, 6900 Heidelberg, FRG

Paul Hermanek, M.D., Professor, Department of Surgical Pathology, University of Erlangen, 8520 Erlangen, FRG

Arnulf H. Hölscher, M.D., Department of Surgery, Technical University of Munich, Klinikum Rechts des Isar, 8000 Munich, FRG

Jürgen Hotz, M.D., Professor of Medicine, Head, Department of Gastroenterology and Oncology, General Hospital, 3100 Celle, FRG

J. Jähne, M.D., Center for Surgery, Medical University of Hannover, 3000 Hannover, FRG

Peter Langhans, M.D., Professor of Surgery, Surgical Clinic and Policlinic of the Westf. Wilhelms University, 4400 Münster, FRG

Hans-Joachim Meyer, M.D., Professor of Surgery, Department of Surgery, Division of Abdominal and Transplantation Surgery, Medical University of Hannover, 3000 Hannover, FRG

H. Milbradt, M.D., Section of Radiologic Diagnostics, Center for Radiology, Medical University of Hannover, 3000 Hannover, FRG

R. Pichlmayr, M.D., Professor, Clinic for Abdominal and Transplantation Surgery, Central Clinic, 3000 Hannover, FRG

H. Poliwoda, M.D., Department of Surgery, Division of Medical Oncology, University of Münster, 4400 Münster, FRG

Peter W. Preusser, M.D., Ph.D., Department of Surgery, Division of Medical Oncology, University of Münster, 4400 Münster, FRG

Wolfgang Rösch, M.D., Professor of Medicine, Head, Department of Medicine, Northwest Hospital, 6000 Frankfurt, FRG

Peter Schlag, M.D., Professor of Surgical Oncology, Department of Surgery, University of Heidelberg, 6900 Heidelberg, FRG

H.-J. Schmoll, M.D., Professor, Department of Hematology/Oncology, Medical University of Hannover, 3000 Hannover, FRG

G. Schüder, M.D., Surgical University Clinic, 6650 Homburg/Saar, FRG

M. Schüler, M.D., Department of Surgery, Technical University of Munich, Klinikum Rechts des Isar, 8000 Munich, FRG

J.R. Siewert, M.D., Professor, Surgical Clinic Rechts der Isar, 8000 Munich, FRG

Hansjochen Wilke, M.D., Associate Professor, Department of Hematology/Oncology, Medical University of Hannover, 3000 Hannover, FRG

J.A. Wils, M.D., Ph.D., Laurentius Hospital, 6043 Roermund, The Netherlands

Abbreviations

ADM	doxorubicin (Adriamycin)
Ara-C	cytosine arabinoside
AJCC	American Joint Committee on Cancer
AP	alkaline phosphatase
BAFMi	BCNU/ADM/5-FU/MTC
BCNU	carmustine
CBC	complete blood count
cCR	clinically complete remission
CDDP	cisplatin
CEA	carcinoembryonic antigen
cPR	clinically partial remission
CNS	central nervous system
CR	complete remission
CT	computerized tomography
EAP	etoposide/ADM/CDDP
Epi-ADM	epidoxorubicin
FA	5-FU/ADM
FAM	5-FU/ADM/MTC
FAMB	5-FU/ADM/BCNU
FAMe	5-FU/ADM/MeCCNU
FAMMe	5-FU/ADM/MTC/MeCCNU
FAMTX	5-FU/ADM/MTX
FAP	5-FU/ADM/CDDP
FMC	5-FU/MTC/Ara-C
FMe	5-FU/MeCCNU
GITSG	Gastrointestinal Tumor Study Group
IFN	interferon
IP	intraperitoneal
IV	intravenous
LV	leukovorin
MeCCNU	semustine

MOF	MTC/vincristine/5-FU
MTC	mitomycin C
NED	no evidence of disease
MTX	methotrexate
NMR	nuclear magnetic resonance
PR	partial remission
TSPA	Triethylenethiophosphoramide
TZT	triazinate

Part I
Pathogenesis and Pathology of Gastric Carcinoma

CHAPTER 1

Epidemiology and Pathogenesis of Gastric Carcinoma

J. Hotz and H. Goebell

Introduction

Worldwide studies on the epidemiology of gastric carcinoma are helping us to understand the correlations between possible causal and risk factors and the development of gastric cancer. Remarkable findings include the very different incidences in various countries and continents, the lack of important hereditary and ethnic factors, and the identification of specific risk factors, especially eating habits and other environmental influences. Knowing the epidemiology of gastric carcinoma also contributes to an understanding of pathogenesis. While these obvious correlations do not constitute proof in most cases, they do provide the data and impetus for controlled scientific, clinical, and experimental studies. It therefore makes sense to review the currently valid facts and speculations about the epidemiology and pathogenesis of gastric carcinoma before discussing the practical and clinical aspects involved in its classification, diagnosis, and therapy. In addition to internationally published results (essentially from the study group of Correa and Pfeiffer) we discuss current epidemiologic data, especially those relating to the incidence in the Federal Republic of Germany, based on the mortality rate statistics of the Federal Office of Statistics and the cancer atlas of the Federal Republic of Germany.[1]

Incidence and Its Development

The incidence and mortality rate statistics of gastric carcinoma indicate a clear decline in almost all countries and continents. This trend is particularly strong in the Western industrialized countries but may also be detected to a somewhat lesser extent in Eastern Europe and other regions.[1] A particularly strong decrease in incidence was already observed to occur in the United States from 1935 to 1960.[2] Even the trend is downward, incidence rates are the highest in Japan, with over 100 new cases per year for every 100,000 inhabitants, and in South America, especially Chile.

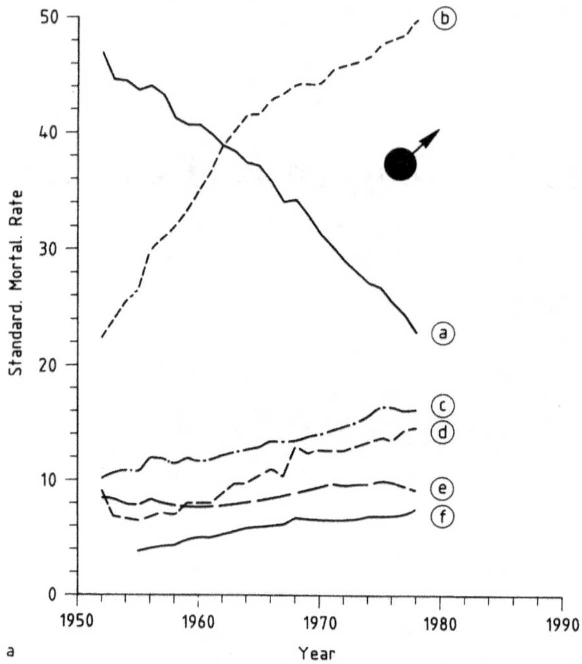

Fig. 1. Trend in age-standardized mortality rates for six types of cancer over time. (**A**) Men: a, stomach; b, lung; c, prostate; d, colon; e, rectum; f, pancreas. (**B**) Women: a, stomach; b, breast; c, uterine fundus; d, colon; e, rectum; f, lung. Reprinted from ref. 1, with permission.

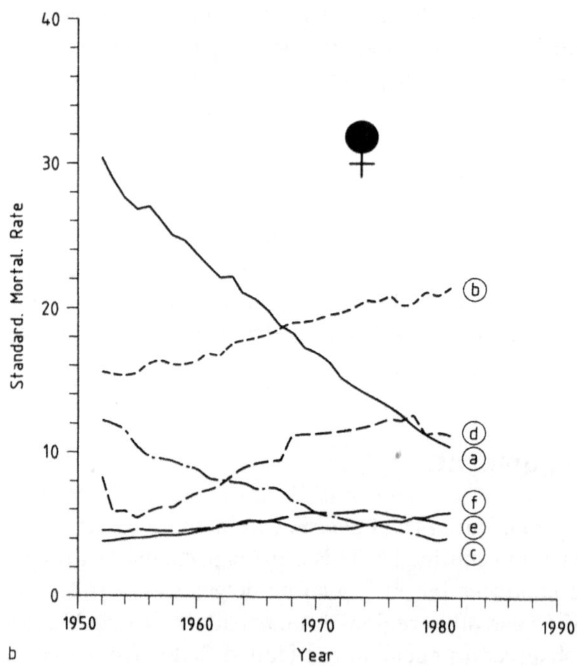

Most cases of gastric carcinoma occur in men (ratio of approximately 2:1), particularly in countries with the highest incidences. Incidence rates reported in Yugoslavia, Rumania, and Poland are especially high—between 25 and 45 cases per 100,000 inhabitants every year. Notably low incidence rates—10 or fewer cases per 100,000 inhabitants—are found in Anglo-American regions. Incidence in the Federal Republic of Germany is intermediate. This statement must be qualified, however; with the exception of individual small states such as Hamburg and Saarland,[1] only mortality statistics are available for the Federal Republic of Germany.

Since the mortality and prognosis of gastric carcinoma have decreased only negligibly in the last two decades, with an average 5-year survival rate of less than 15%, it is admissible to draw conclusions about individual incidences from the mortality-rate statistics, especially when assessing the changes in incidences over time.

The Federal Republic of Germany

In 1980 in the Federal Republic of Germany, gastric carcinoma represented the second most frequent cause of cancer-related deaths after lung cancer among the male population at 11.6%, followed by colon and rectal cancer, prostate cancer, and pancreatic cancer. Among the female population, gastric carcinoma came in third at 9.7% after breast cancer and colorectal carcinoma in the same year.[1] Figures 1A and 1B reveal a highly significant drop in deaths related to gastric carcinoma from 1952 to 1982 for both men and women. Increases in lung cancer incidences in men and breast cancer in women occurred simultaneously. Deaths related to colon carcinoma almost doubled, given a constant rectal cancer mortality rate over this period of time. The drop in the number of deaths due to gastric carcinoma each year in men went from 47 per 100,000 to 20 per 100,000 in the two decades from 1952 to 1982. The latest figures for 1985 put the incidence at 16 per 100,000; the trend has therefore continued in recent years. The overall rate is clearly lower for women, with a drop from approximately 30 deaths per 100,000 inhabitants each year in 1952 to below 10 in 1982. As in other countries, a cohort phenomenon may be observed in the Federal Republic of Germany, ie, the younger generations clearly exhibit a lower overall decrease in the number of deaths due to gastric carcinoma compared with the older populations. Figure 2 illustrates this varying trend toward decreases in cohorts of birth spaced at 5-year intervals. The trend is more pronounced in older patients aged 60 to 64 years than in the younger cohorts by birth. We may assume from this that possible risk factors may have had particularly strong effects during the youth of the pre-1920 cohorts. Older generations consequently have a higher risk of developing gastric carcinoma compared with earlier generations, where the development of gastric carcinoma was evidently prevented in part by factors still to be identified in greater detail.

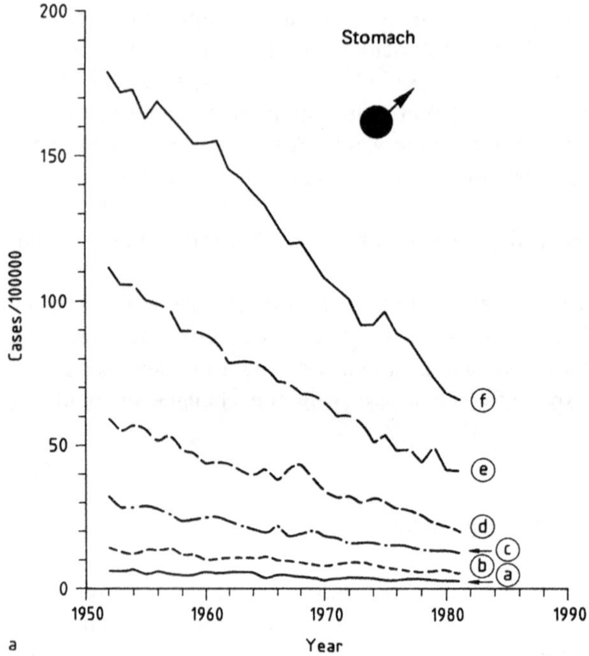

a

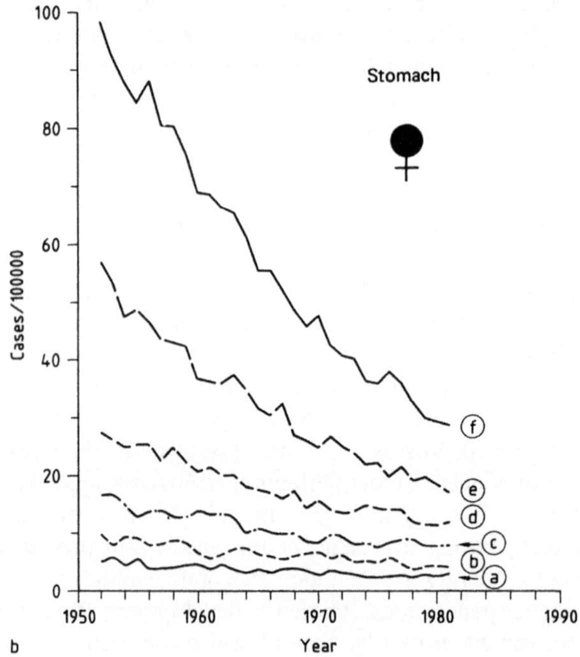

b

Fig. 2. Trend in mortality rate for individual age groups over time. (**A**) Men: a, 35–39; b, 40–44; c, 45–49; d, 50–54; e, 55–59; f, 60–64. (**B**) Women: a, 35–39; b, 40–44; c, 45–49; d, 50–54; e, 55–59; f, 60–64. Reprinted from ref. 1, with permission.

Mortality-rate statistics for gastric carcinoma reveal considerable geographic differences in the Federal Republic of Germany, with a distinct concentration in Bavaria (over 28.5 per 100,000 for men and 15 per 100,000 for women in 1978) and North Rhine–Westphalia and parts of Lower Saxony (24–28 and 12–15 per 100,000), while incidence rates were often lower in adjacent regions such as Hessen and Swabia at under 20 and 10 per 100,000 (all figures for 1978).[1] Possible nutritional and environmental factors will be considered in the next section.

It may be concluded for the Federal Republic of Germany that death due to gastric carcinoma, and hence the incidence in both sexes, is decreasing while remaining predominant in men, with regional differences retained.

Studies in Immigrants

The literature provides numerous indications that the largely disparate global and regional incidence of gastric carcinoma may be more attributable to environmental influences than to ethnic, racial, or genetic factors. Environmental factors are probably most relevant in the first two to three decades of life, according to so-called immigrant studies.[3,4] Considerable differences between incidence rates for the countries of origin and immigration can be found among immigrants and their children. This is demonstrated most strikingly in the case of immigrants coming to the United States from countries with a high risk for the disease, such as Japan, Poland, and Iceland. These immigrants have a high risk for gastric carcinoma similar as that in the country of origin, while the first- and especially the second-generation descendants exhibit increasingly lower incidence rates which approach that of the United States population as a whole.

Habs and Schmähl[5] contrasted the risk for gastric carcinoma in Japanese immigrants and two succeeding generations against the risk for colon cancer (Fig. 3). While the incidences for both kinds of tumors in these immigrants were similar in their country of origin (Japan), the risk of developing gastric carcinoma decreased as the risk of colon cancer increased.

Are There Two Epidemiologically Different Tumor Types?

The literature suggests that countries with a high incidence rate (especially Japan) have an overall considerably lower mortality rate for gastric carcinoma (approximately 50%) compared with countries that have a low incidence rate, such as the Federal Republic of Germany and the United States, where the mortality rate is estimated to be higher than 80%.

Prognosis may thus depend on the type of gastric carcinoma. The more common type is caused by early exogenous factors that lead to a more favorable prognostic course; the less common type has less of an environmental etiology and a poorer prognosis. Early studies in Finland by Laurén and associates had already

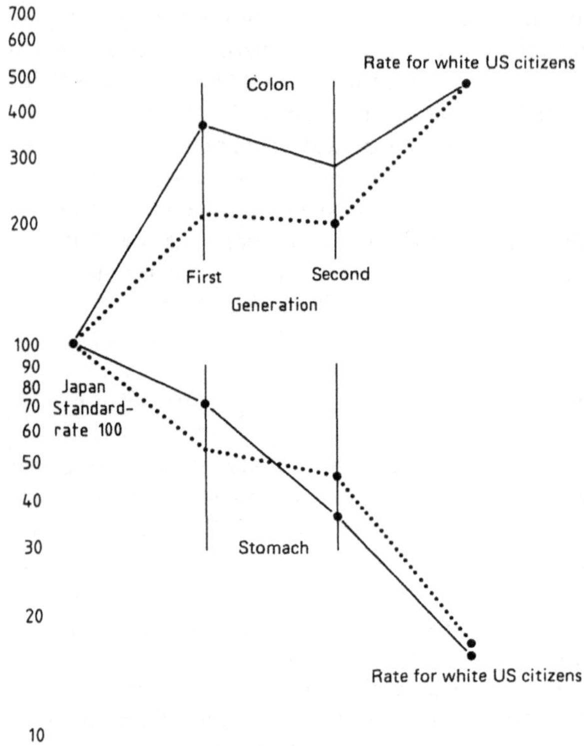

Fig. 3. Trend in mortality rate for gastric and colon cancer in Japanese immigrants to the United States over two generations. (Reprinted from Habs M, Schmähl D: Karzinogene Substanzen in der Nahrung. Inn Med 1979;6:237, with permission of Pflaum Verlag München.)

indicated the existence of two morphologically different types, whose basic difference has to do with the extent to which the cells in the tumor belong together.[6,7] The intestinal type of tumor retains sufficient cell cohesion forming gland-like tubular structures, while the diffuse type has no cell cohesion and is characterized by infiltration into the subepithelial intramural structures. Due to the differing mode of propagation, the terms "expansive" and "infiltrative" were suggested for the intestinal and diffuse types, respectively.[8] Epidemiologic studies demonstrated that the intestinal, expansive type may be encountered especially in countries having a high incidence of gastric carcinoma, which is the reason that this type was also designated as epidemic. In contrast, the incidence rate for the diffuse, infiltrative type of tumor is similarly high in most populations, and for this reason was designated as endemic.[9] Also notable is that the worldwide drop in gastric carcinoma observed over the last decades essentially may be traced back to a reduction in the intestinal, expansive, epidemic type. All of these observations lead to the conclusion that environmental factors play an important pathogenetic role for this cell type, and that any changes in these factors can result in a change in the risk associated with this type of tumor. Other epidemiologic characteristics of both types of gastric carcinoma are summarized in Table 1.

Table 1. Characteristics of gastric carcinoma by histological type[a]

Intestinal (expansive)	Diffuse (infiltrative)
Epidemic	Endemic
Men > Women	Women > Men
Older	Younger
Increased incidence +	Increased incidence −
Decreased incidence +	Decreased incidence −
Prognosis: Relatively good	Prognosis: Poor
Precancerous +	Precancerous − (?)
Familial predisposition (blood group) −	Familial predisposition (blood group) +

[a] Laurén P: The two histological main types of gastric carcinoma: diffuse and so-called intestinal-type carcinoma: an attempt at a histoclinical classification. *Acta Pathol Microbiol Scand* 1965;64:31. Reprinted with permission.

The intestinal, expansive, epidemic type is encountered primarily in men older than 60 years. The prognosis is relatively favorable, and precancerous stages which may lead to a carcinoma of this type can be identified (see below). Familial predisposition cannot be confirmed. In contrast, the diffuse, infiltrative, endemic type shows no preference for either sex, and incidence of the disease clearly peaks at a younger age. Interestingly, when viewed in absolute terms, the diffuse tumor type does not occur more frequently in countries with a higher incidence of gastric carcinoma. Prognosis for the often relatively young patients is decidedly poor.

A recent publication from Tso and associates in Correa's group[10] confirms this: 38 of 1,710 patients with gastric carcinoma studied from 1948 to 1983 were younger than 35 years. Distribution by sex was the same, and the diffuse, scirrhous infiltrative type predominated histologically. Even though tumor could be resected almost as often as in the higher age groups, the prognosis was poor—only 1 of the 38 patients survived for a full 5 years. Other authors report similar experiences.[6,11] A familial predisposition (ie, via predominance of blood group A) could be determined for the diffuse type, while precancerous stages have not yet been established for this type.[9]

Environmental Factors: Nutrition

Even though we still have no proof that certain environmental factors—especially dietary influences—predispose to the development of gastric carcinoma, the varying worldwide distribution of gastric carcinoma leads us to assume that different environmental factors may at least play a permissive role in the pathogenetic chain of development. In particular, neighboring, ethnically similar, populations have different incidences of gastric carcinoma when cultural and not ethnic differences exist. On the other hand, differences in the eating habits of populations of various continents having a similar risk of developing the disease clearly exist.

Table 2. Environmental and nutritional factors that facilitate the development (risk factors) or reduce the risk (protective factors) of gastric carcinoma

Risk factors	Protective factors
Low consumption of fat/protein	Foods rich in vitamins C and A
Grains	Fresh vegetables/fruit
Salts (salted meat/fish)	High protein/fat consumption (?)
Nitrates (drinking water)	Deep-freeze preservation
Low consumption of salad, vegetables, fruit	Careful food preparation
Fava beans	Better drinking water supply
Smoked meats (ham, fish)	

A comparative study failed to identify any specific substance or foodstuff, instead bringing to light a certain pattern of nutrition observed primarily in countries with an elevated risk of stomach cancer. The eating habits in countries having a typically low risk of disease were simultaneously introduced as protective factors (Table 2). According to these studies, high-risk nutrition is characterized by a low proportion of animal fat and protein, together with a high proportion of hard-to-digest carbohydrates, highly salted foods, especially salted meats and fish, a high proportion of smoked meats and fish, a high proportion of fava beans, and a strikingly low proportion of salads, vegetables, and fruits. In agreement with the above, the protective factors in countries with a low incidence of carcinoma, in particular the United States, include a diet rich in vitamin C and vitamin A with a high proportion of fresh vegetables and fruit as well as high consumption of proteins and fat. The nitration of drinking water was also addressed as an important cause for the development of gastric carcinoma, especially after a reduction in the risk was observed following the switch to a more modern drinking water supply.[12-14] The drop in the incidence of gastric carcinoma in Japan was similarly correlated to a reduction in pickled meat and the introduction of more refrigerators.[15]

Elevated consumption of alcohol and nicotine is also considered a risk factor for the development of gastric carcinoma.[16] Increased incidence of gastric carcinoma was found in coal miners who had been exposed to coal dust for long periods of time and who simultaneously smoked a large number of cigarettes.[17,18] Increased exposure to asbestos, however, does not appear to be associated with higher risk.[19] This is important because the elevated rate of gastric carcinoma in Japan had at one time been correlated with the increased consumption of rice contaminated by asbestos, among other factors. Also, the fact that other countries that consume large quantities of rice, such as India, tend to have a low incidence of gastric carcinoma casts further doubt on the "rice hypothesis."[4]

Pathogenesis

The pathogenesis of the diffuse, infiltrative-scirrhous type of gastric carcinoma is unclear. Data concerning premalignant lesions are lacking. In contrast, the intestinal type appears to be the final result of a series of mutations and cell transformations.[20] Certain types of chronic gastritis may be viewed as an early stage of this process. Also termed hypersecretory, simple chronic superficial gastritis or chronic-atrophic gastritis with pylorocardial spreading primarily restricted to the antrum does not appear to play an important role here. The autoimmune type A gastritis, which is limited to the corpus, is a more likely precancerous stage. Correa[21] introduced the concept of "environmentally induced" chronic gastritis as a third possible type of gastritis which may in turn be viewed as a precancerous stage. Environmentally induced gastritis is characterized by a multifocal circumscribed distribution in the antrum and corpus, most probably at the corpus-antrum junction during early stages. The gastritic changes are typically accompanied by atrophy, intestinal metaplasia, and occasional dysplasia of the gastric mucosa in type A gastritis as well as in environmentally induced gastritis. In contrast, chronic-atrophic gastritis appears in cluster form during a peptic ulceration where atrophy represents the final stage of the gastritic changes. Atrophy is therefore apparently the important link in the development of gastritis to mucosal neoplasia. The possible stages of development are diagrammed in Figure 4.

Type A gastritis or environmentally induced chronic gastritis leads to mucosal atrophy with the formation of either intestinal metaplasia or dysplasia. Intestinal metaplasia—the transformation of the cells of the gastric mucosa—may proceed in either of two ways. Mature cells resembling enterocytes with a stock of enzymes comparable to the epithelia of the small intestine arise (this type of cell exhibits no tendency toward malignant degeneration), or immature intestinal cells develop with the typical stock of enzymes having been lost. Such a form of intestinal metaplasia with immature cell colonies exhibits a tendency toward

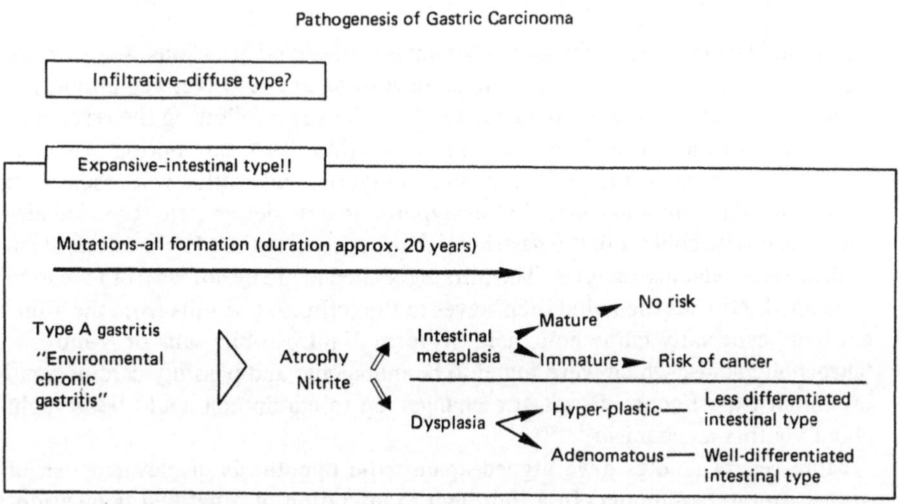

Fig. 4. Pathogenesis of gastric carcinoma classified by diffuse and intestinal type, according to Laurén. (Reprinted from Correa P: Carcinoma of the stomach. Proc Nutr Soc 1985;44:111, with permission of Cambridge University Press.)

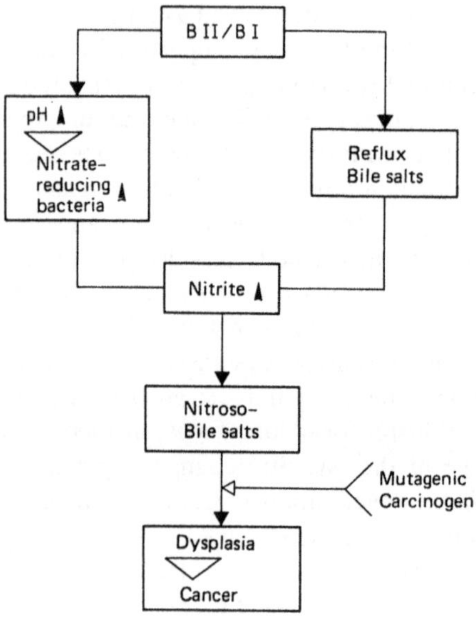

Fig. 5. Pathnogenesis of postoperative carcinoma after gastric resection (Billroth I and II). Hypothetical model.

malignant degeneration. Hyperplastic and adenomatous dysplasias may be distinguished when an atrophy develops into dysplasia. Both changes are to be regarded as precancerous (cf. the paper of Hermanek for more specifics on pathogenesis).

Partial Gastrectomy as a Precancerous Stage?

An elevated cancer risk in the gastric stump was observed in various studies more than 15 years after Billroth II resections. According to a 1971 Norwegian study,[22] relative risk rose from 5 to 10 during the 15 to 35 years following the resection, compared with a risk of 1 in a normal population. This assumption was confirmed in subsequent studies.[22] As shown in Figure 5, bile reflux was assumed to be pathogenetically important. In this hypothetical model, gastric resection elevates the nitrite content in the gastric juice by increasing the pH via colonization with nitrate-reducing bacteria. The nitrate reduced to nitrite comes from the food consumed. Nitrites then bind themselves to the refluxed bile salts from the afferent loop, especially taurocholic acid, to form *N*-nitroso-bile salts or *N*-nitroso-taurocholic acids, which were found to be mutagenic and possibly carcinogenic in animal experiments. Dysplastic changes up to carcinoma could be brought about via this mechanism.[23–25]

More recent studies have argued against the hypothesis of elevated risk of gastric stump carcinoma. In a thorough examination of a defined population, Schafter and associates[26] were unable to find an elevated risk of stump carcinoma in 338 patients who had undergone partial gastric resections from 1935 to 1959 due to gastroduodenal ulcers. Only two cases of stump carcinoma were discovered. In another prospective study done in Japan, a lower than normal incidence of gastric carcinoma was found in 387 patients during a 10-year and longer follow-up period.[27] Another negative study which also failed to turn up an elevated incidence of carcinoma in the residual stomach was reported in the United States. In contrast, an earlier retrospective study from Italy reported an increase in the overall risk for gastric stump carcinoma following Billroth I and II operations.[28] Interestingly, cholecystectomy is not associated with a higher risk of gastric carcinoma after an interval of over 15 years.[29] The fact that the peak age of patients with gastric stump carcinoma is about as high as that of individuals with an intact stomach also speaks against a causal relationship. In addition, the relative distribution of the intestinal and diffuse types is similar in postoperative carcinoma as in carcinomas of the intact stomach (P. Hermanek, 1987, personal communication). Exogenous factors such as elevated alcohol and nicotine consumption probably play a part in the incidence of clustered carcinoma in the gastric stump observed in several studies.

Conclusions

The most important epidemiologic and pathogenetic data regarding gastric carcinoma lead to the following conclusions. The extremely different incidence of this type of cancer worldwide is more likely caused by varying exposure to certain environmental factors than by ethnic, genetic, or racial differences. The intestinal, expansive type is histologically more frequent among high-risk populations, with a preference for men and older individuals, and a more favorable prognosis than the diffuse type. In contrast, a relatively more frequent diffuse, infiltrative histological type is typical of populations at lower risk of gastric cancer, with a slight preference for women and younger patients and a poorer prognosis. Presumed to be decisive environmental factors which probably determine the higher risk of gastric carcinoma in later years are nutritional loads to the gastric mucosa in the first two to three decades of life. Highly salted and smoked meals, diets rich in grains but poor in vitamin C, and food preservation with nitrites are regarded as causal factors. Precancerous conditions in high-risk populations might be certain kinds of atrophic gastritis or intestinal metaplasia, while recent studies cast doubt on any risk for gastric stump carcinoma following Billroth I or II operations.

Certain clinically relevant conclusions may be drawn from these data. Specific nutritional guidelines, such as eating foods low in salt and rich in vitamin C, staying away from smoked meals and artificial preservation (eg, with nitrites), and using unprocessed, unpreserved foods, must be followed to reduce the risk of gastric carcinoma in a given population. In addition, risk groups should be given routine follow-up examinations, as should patients with detected dysplasia and other precancerous lesions. Not enough research has focused on the correlations, particularly between the degree of dysplasia and the development of gastric carcinoma. Controlled, long-term scientific studies are therefore necessary, especially with regard to this question.

References

1. Becker N, Frentzel-Beyme R, Wagner G: Krebsatlas der BRD, 2 ed. Berlin-Heidelberg-New York, Springer, 1984, p 50.
2. Higginson J: Worldwide review of epidemiology of gastric cancer, in Hirayama T (ed): Epidemiology of Stomach Cancer: Key Questions and Answers. WHO CC, monograph, 1977, p. 81.
3. Haenszel WM: Cancer mortality and incidence among the foreign born in the United States. J Natl Cancer Inst 1961;26:37.
4. Naujoks-Heinrich S, Dölle W: Die Epidemiologie der häufigsten Tumoren des Verdauungskanals. Internist 1982;23:1.
5. Habs M, Schmähl D: Karzinogene Substanzen in der Nahrung. Inn Med 1979;6:237.
6. Grabiec J, Owen DA: Carcinoma of the stomach in young persons. Cancer 1985; 56:388.
7. Laurén P: The two histological main types of gastric carcinoma: diffuse and so-called intestinal-type carcinoma: an attempt at a histoclinical classification. Acta Pathol Microbiol Scand 1965;64:31.
8. Muñoz N, Connelly R: Time trends of intestinal and diffuse types of gastric cancer in the United States. Int J Cancer 1971;8:158.
9. Correa P, Sasano N, Stemmermann GN, et al: Pathology of gastric carcinoma in Japanese populations: comparison between Miyagi Prefecture, Japan and Hawaii. J Natl Cancer Inst 1973;51:1449.
10. Tso PL, Bringaze III WL, Dauterive AH, et al: Gastric carcinoma in the young. Cancer 1987;59:1362.
11. Mori M, Sugimachi K, Ohiwa T, et al: Early gastric carcinoma in Japanese patients under 30 years of age. Br J Surg 1985;72:289.
12. Cuello C, Correa P, Haenszel W, et al: Gastric cancer in Colombia: cancer risk and suspected environmental agents. J Natl Cancer Inst 1976;57:1015.
13. Fraser P, Chilvers C, Beral V, et al: Nitrate and human cancer: a review of the evidence. Int J Epidemiol 1980;9:3.
14. Correa P, Haenszel W, Tannenbaum S: Epidemiology of gastric carcinoma. Natl Cancer Inst Monogr 1982;62:129.
15. Hirayama T: Epidemiology of stomach cancer in Japan with special reference to strategy for the primary prevention. Jap J Clin Oncol 1984;14:159.
16. Correa P, Fontham E, Pickle LW, et al: Dietary determinants of gastric cancer in South Louisiana inhabitants. J Natl Cancer Inst 1985;75:645.
17. Ames RG: Gastric cancer and coal mine dust exposure: a case control study. Cancer 1983;52:1346.
18. Matolo NM, Klauber MR, Gorishek WM, et al: High incidence of gastric carcinoma in a coal mining region. Cancer 1972;29:733.
19. Neuberger M, Kundi M, Friodl HP: Environmental asbestos exposure and cancer mortality. Arch Environ Health 1984;39:261.
20. Correa P, Haenszel W, Cuello C, et al: A model for gastric cancer epidemiology. Lancet 1975;2:58.

21. Correa P: The epidemiology and pathogenesis of chronic gastritis: three etiologic entities. Front Gastroenterol Res 1980;6:98.
22. Nichols JC: Stump cancer following gastric surgery. World J Surg 1979;3:731.
23. Dahm K, Werner B, Mitschke H: Experimental cancer of the gastric stump, in Herfarth C, Schlag P (eds): Gastric Cancer. Berlin-Heidelberg-New York, Springer, 1979, p 44.
24. Langhans P, Heger RA, Hobenstein F, et al: Operation sequel carcinoma. An experimental study. Hepatogastroenterology 1981;28:34.
25. Schlag P, Bockler R, Meyer H, et al: Nitrite and N-nitrosocompounds in the operated stomach, in Herfarth C, Schlag P (eds): Gastric Cancer, Berlin-Heidelberg-New York, Springer, 1979, p 120.
26. Schafter LW, Larson DE, Melton III LS, et al: The risk of gastric carcinoma after surgical treatment for benign ulcer disease: a population-based study in Olmstead County, Minnesota. N Engl J Med 1983;309:1210.
27. Tokudome S, Suminori K, Masato I, et al: A prospective study on primary gastric stump cancer following partial gastrectomy for benign gastroduodenal diseases. Cancer Res 1984;44:2208.
28. Giarelli L, Melato M, Stanta G, et al: Gastric resection: a cause of high frequency of gastric carcinoma. Cancer 1983;52:1113.
29. Gustavsson S, Adami HO, Meirik O, et al: Cholecystectomy as a risk factor for gastric cancer: a cohort study. Dig Dis Sci 1984;29:116.

CHAPTER 2

Gastric Carcinoma—Precancerous Conditions and Lesions, Classification, and Prognosis

P. Hermanek

Precancerous Conditions and Lesions

As has been done for other organs, the term "precancerosis" with regard to the stomach should be subdivided into two separate categories. A *precancerous condition* is a clinically defined state which involves an elevated risk of cancer in comparison with the normal population. By contrast, a *precancerous lesion* is defined as a histopathologic abnormality in which cancer is more likely to occur than its apparently normal counterpart. Epithelial dysplasia is the histological substrate of the precancerous lesion.[1]

The main problem associated with precancerous conditions and lesions in the stomach is that the two primary histological types of gastric carcinomas—what Laurén calls intestinal and diffuse—differ epidemiologically and pathogenetically. In addition, our knowledge about precancerous conditions and lesions essentially relates only to the intestinal type, and we can make no firm and binding statements about diffuse carcinoma.

Precancerous Conditions

Chronic atrophic gastritis with intestinal metaplasia may be viewed primarily as a precancerous condition existing in the stomach. It is generally accompanied by other conditions such as pernicious anemia, polyps in the stomach, and the condition following gastric resection (Fig. 1).

Intestinal metaplasia with a high proportion of sulfomucins primarily appears to be connected with carcinoma,[2–4] and is referred to as incomplete intestinal metaplasia by the WHO classification[5] and enterocolic type of intestinal metaplasia according to Heilmann.[2]

Precancerous conditions also include all clinical situations in which the risk of cancer is generally elevated, such as, for example, corresponding family histories, association with so-called cancer families, acanthosis nigricans, and dermatomyositis.

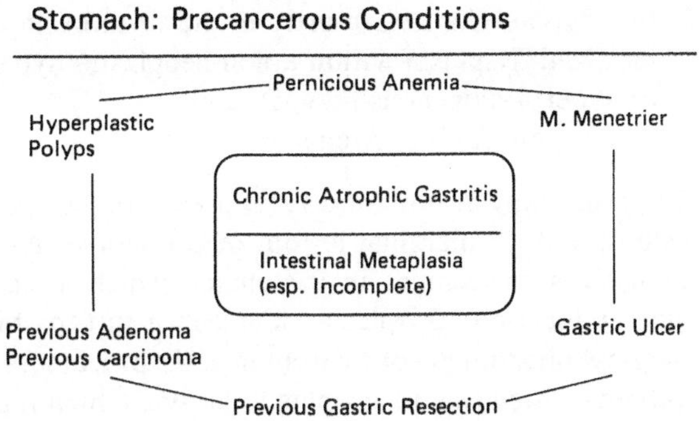

Fig. 1. Overview of precancerous conditions in the stomach.

Precancerous Lesions

As is the case in other sites of the gastrointestinal tract, precancerous lesions in the stomach are characterized histologically by epithelial dysplasia (Fig. 2). Three forms are recognized in the stomach:

1. In flat mucosa, particularly in cases of chronic atrophic gastritis with intestinal metaplasia (especially incomplete) and in the gastric stump, with atrophic gastritis present most of the time as well;

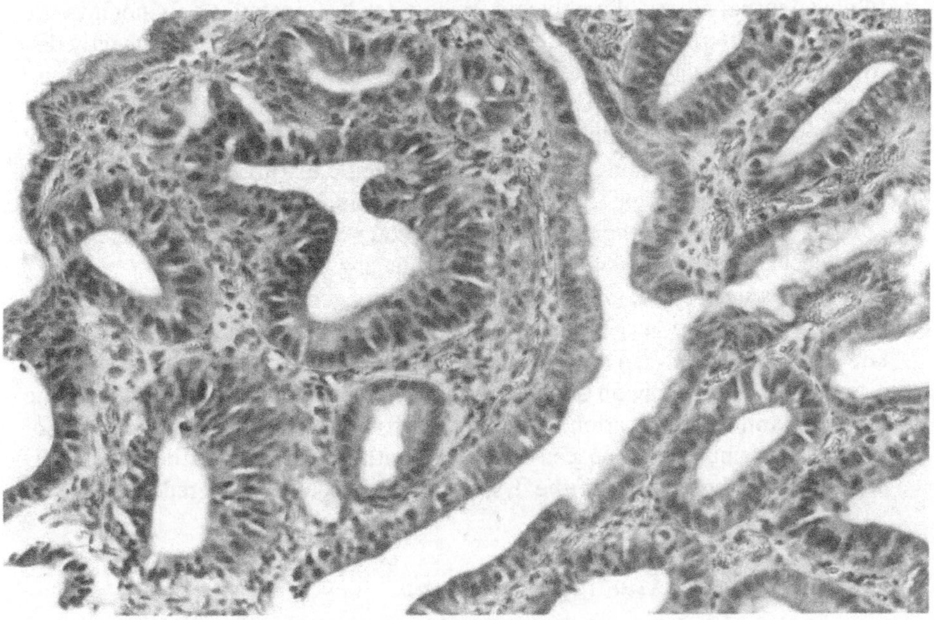

Fig. 2. Polypoid dysplasia of the stomach (chromophotograph).

2. In polypoid changes, mostly in the form of an adenoma and only rarely as localized dysplasia within a non-neoplastic hyperplastic polyp (regenerative or hyperplasiogenous polyps); and
3. In the giant folds of Menetrier's disease.

Dysplasias may be observed as (1) precursor lesions, (2) synchronous associated lesions, and (3) marginal lesions of carcinoma. Associated dysplasias manifest themselves as changes in a stomach which already exhibits a carcinoma in another location. Dysplasias found in a forceps biopsy specimen may be the marginal phenomena of a carcinoma. As precursors, dysplasias are purely intraepithelial, noninvasive neoplastic lesions which may potentially undergo invasive growth at a later point in time, and in so doing trigger transformation into a carcinoma capable of metastasis.

Consequences of Biopsy Diagnosis of Dysplasia

The primary response to a diagnosis of dysplasia obtained by biopsy should be *early repeated gastroscopy.* The goal of the latter procedure is to find any small early carcinoma that may have been overlooked. The job is therefore one of ascertaining that the dysplasia discovered is not a marginal or associated lesion of a carcinoma.

If the *dysplasia was found in a polypoid lesion*, this lesion must be completely removed to eliminate with certainty any carcinoma already present in the polyp. While an initial biopsy of a polypoid lesion often demonstrates only noninvasive epithelial proliferations, a localized invasive carcinoma can be subsequently discovered during examination of the completely removed polypoid lesion. Complete removal may in many cases be accomplished endoscopically. This must otherwise be done surgically by means of a local excision or a distal gastrectomy, depending on the location. These operations should be carried out only in those institutions where intraoperative histological examinations are both possible and reliable. Depending on the findings, the surgical procedure is expanded to a classic cancer operation, if possible performed during the same session.

In cases where *dysplasia is discovered in flat mucosa or giant folds* and even repeated gastroscopy has failed to detect carcinoma in the stomach, a process known as "mapping" is recommended. Multiple topographically characterized biopsies are obtained in an attempt to gain a mental picture of the extent of the dysplasia and its localization. In conclusion, a careful and thorough series of follow-up examinations, spaced 6 to 12 months apart, should be conducted, depending on the severity of the dysplasia (low grade or high grade).

Classification of Gastric Carcinoma

As with tumors in other organs, the classification encompasses both the histomorphology of the tumor as well as the extent of its spread at the time of the diag-

Color Plates

Plate I

Color plates from the chapter by P. Hermanek: Gastric Carcinoma – Precancerous Conditions and Lesions, Classification, and Prognosis

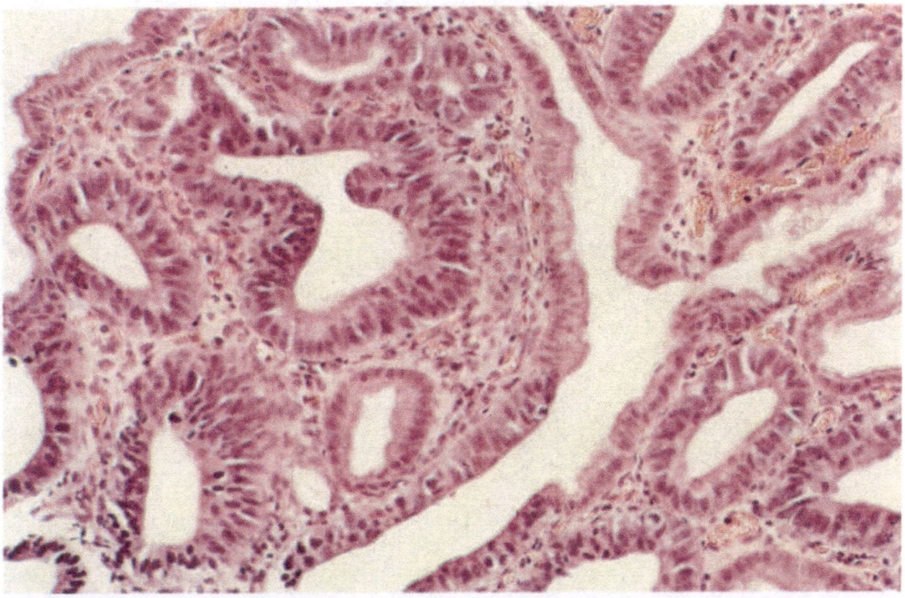

Fig. 2. Polypoid dysplasia of the stomach.

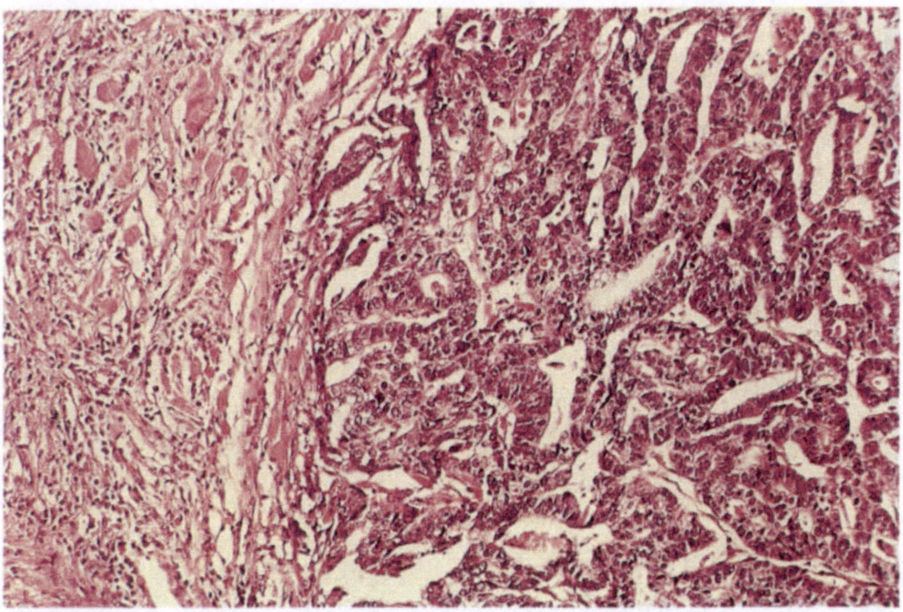

Fig. 3. Gastric carcinoma of intestinal type.

Plate II

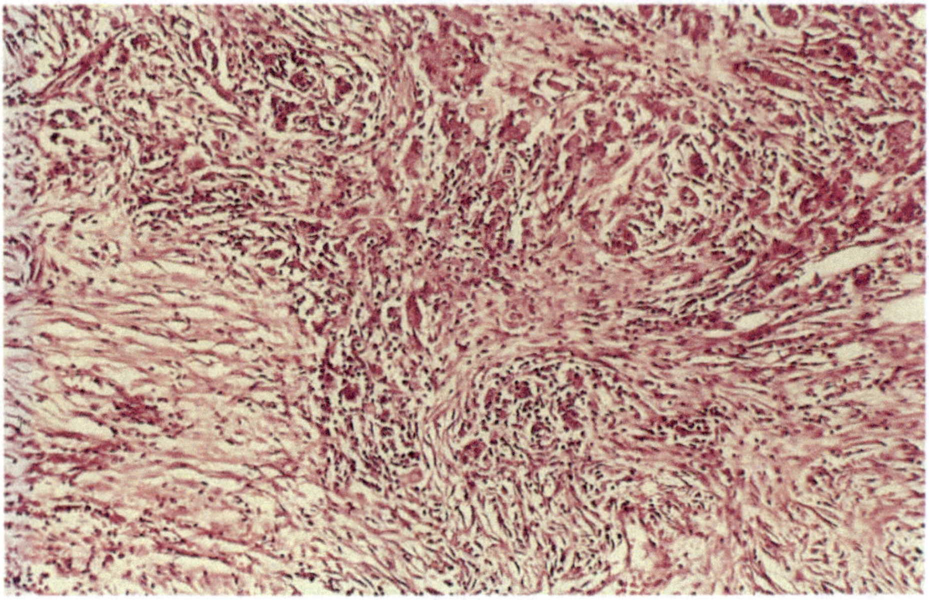

Fig. 4. Gastric carcinoma of diffuse type.

Plate III

Color plates from the chapter by W. Rösch: Endoscopic Criteria for Premalignant Lesions and Early Gastric Carcinoma.

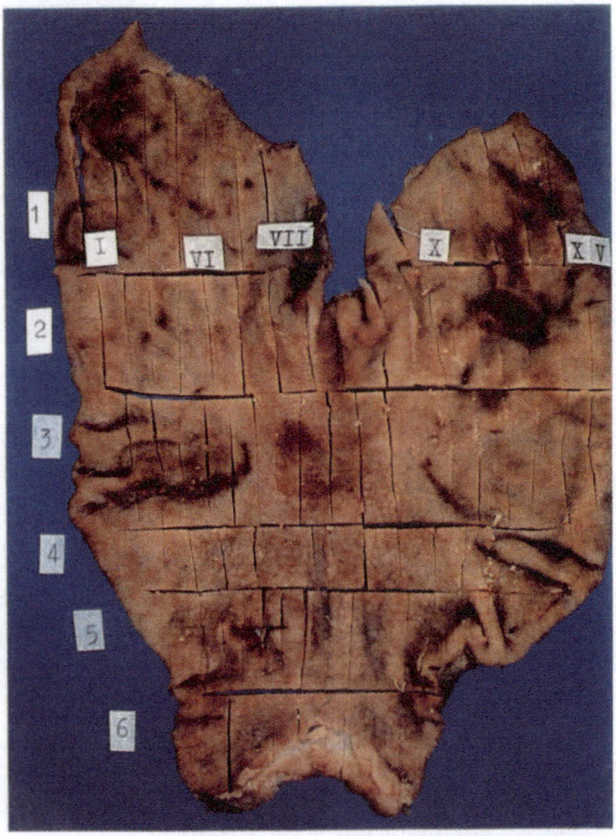

Fig. 2. Histological workup of an early gastric carcinoma.

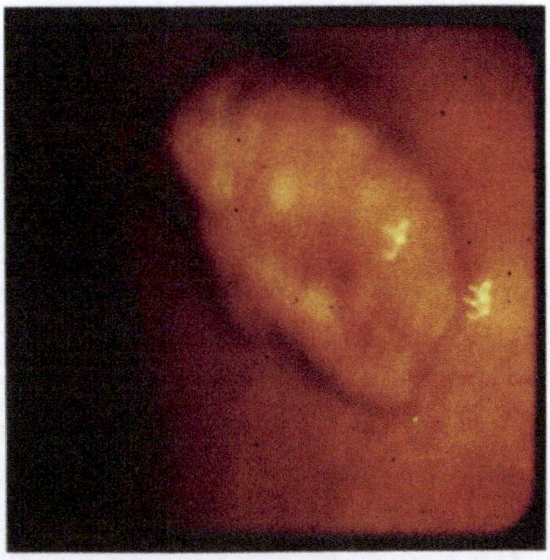

Fig. 3. Early carcinoma, type I.

Plate IV

Fig. 4. Early gastric carcinoma, type IIa.

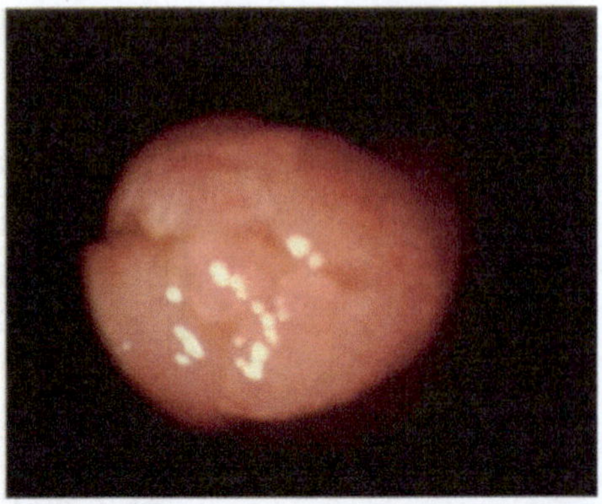

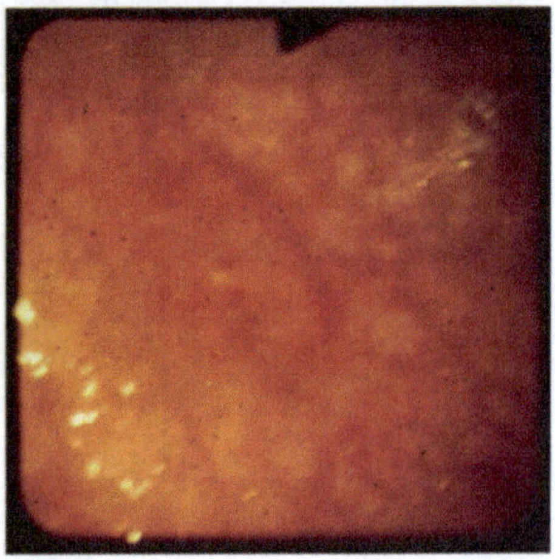

Fig. 5. Early gastric carcinoma, type IIb.

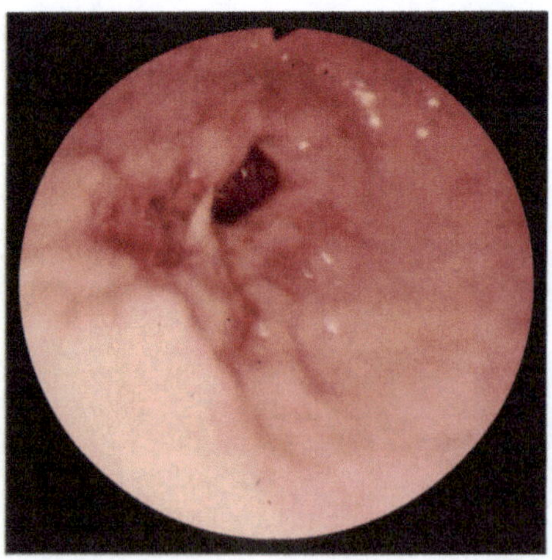

Fig. 6. Early gastric carcinoma, type IIc.

Plate V

Fig. 8. Early gastric carcinoma, type III.

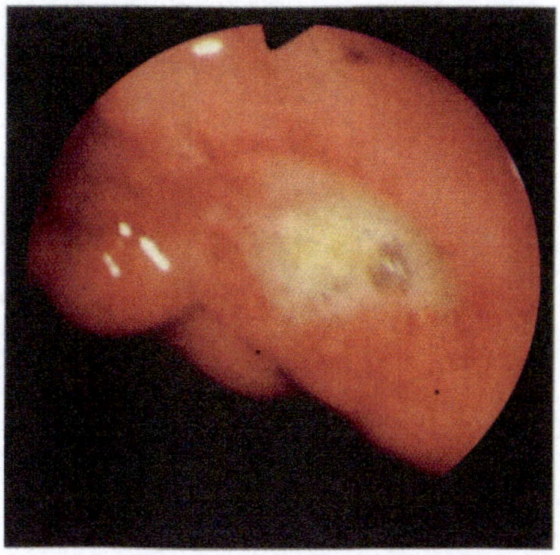

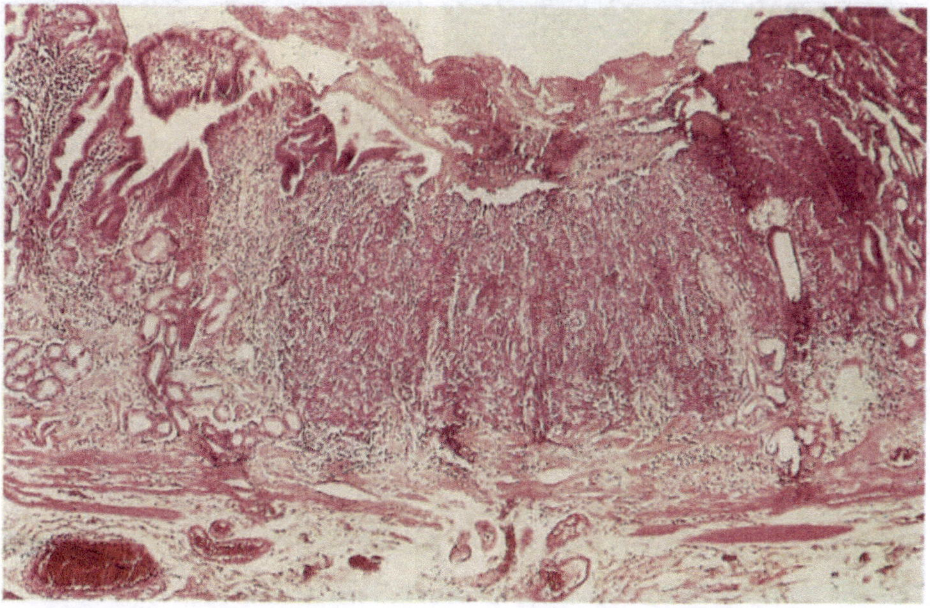

Fig. 10. Early gastric carcinoma 1 × 2 mm in diameter, impressive as erosion.

Plate VI

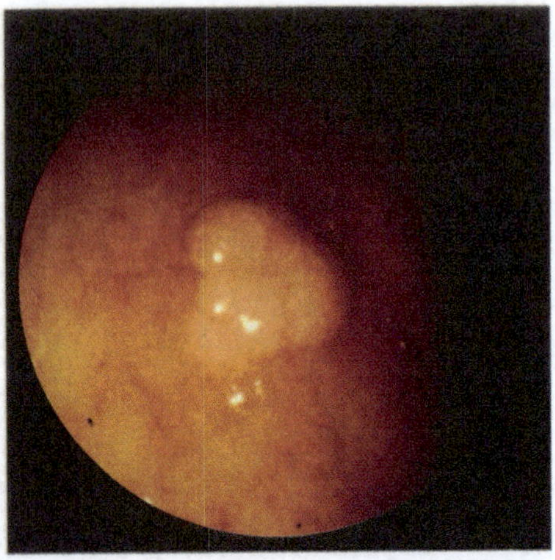

Fig. 11. Adenoma of the gastric mucosa.

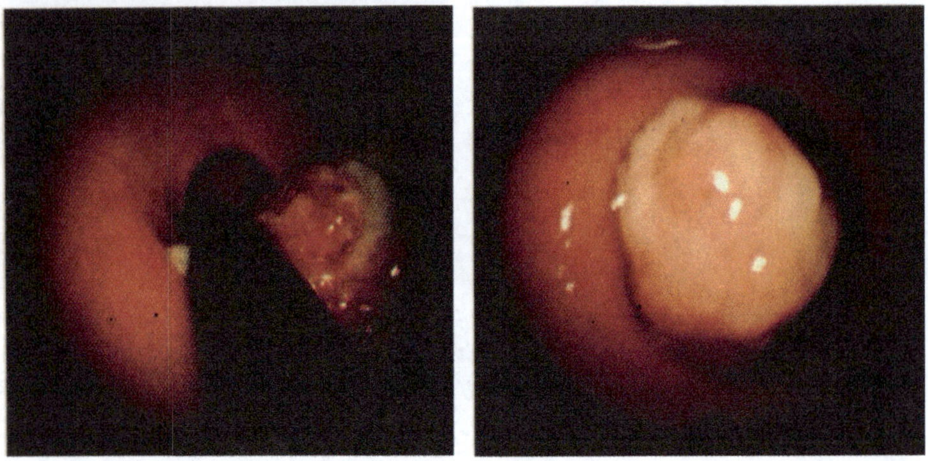

Fig. 12. Borderline lesion, protruded type (flat adenoma).

nosis. The classifications according to WHO and that put together by Laurén are available for categorizing histomorphology (typing and grading). Extent of tumor spread is determined according to the TNM/pTNM system and the stage grouping based upon it (staging).

WHO Classification

According to the WHO classification[6] gastric carcinomas (excluding rarities) are categorized as:

1. Adenocarcinoma
   a. tubular
   b. papillary
   c. mucinous
2. Signet-ring cell carcinoma
3. Undifferentiated carcinoma

Since different structures are often encountered in gastric cancers, the WHO classification explicitly specifies that categories are to be assigned according to the predominant structures. Adenocarcinomas may be further categorized as either well (G1), moderately (G2), or poorly (G3) differentiated. Varying degrees of differentiation often coexist in the one tumor, in which case the WHO

Table 1. Classification of gastric cancer according to Laurén

	Intestinal type	Diffuse type
Histological criteria (= definition)		
Pattern	Primarily glands with cells similar to intestinal columnar cells	Scattered individual cells or small clusters of cells
Demarcation	Mostly sharp	Poor
Cellular cohesion	Good	Bad
Macroscopic pattern	Primarily Borrmann I and II	Primarily Borrmann III and IV
WHO classification	Adenocarcinoma (Gl-3)	Signet-ring cell carcinoma Undifferentiated carcinoma Adenocarcinoma G3
Macroscopic spread to adjacent normal gastric wall (measured in situ)	A few millimeters	Several (up to 8) centimeters
Epidemiology		
Geographic differences in incidence	+++	–
Increased incidence with age	+++	(+)
Predominance of male sex	+++	+
Major etiological factors	Environment	Genetic
Pathogenesis:		
Chronic atrophic gastritis	Almost always	Not inevitable

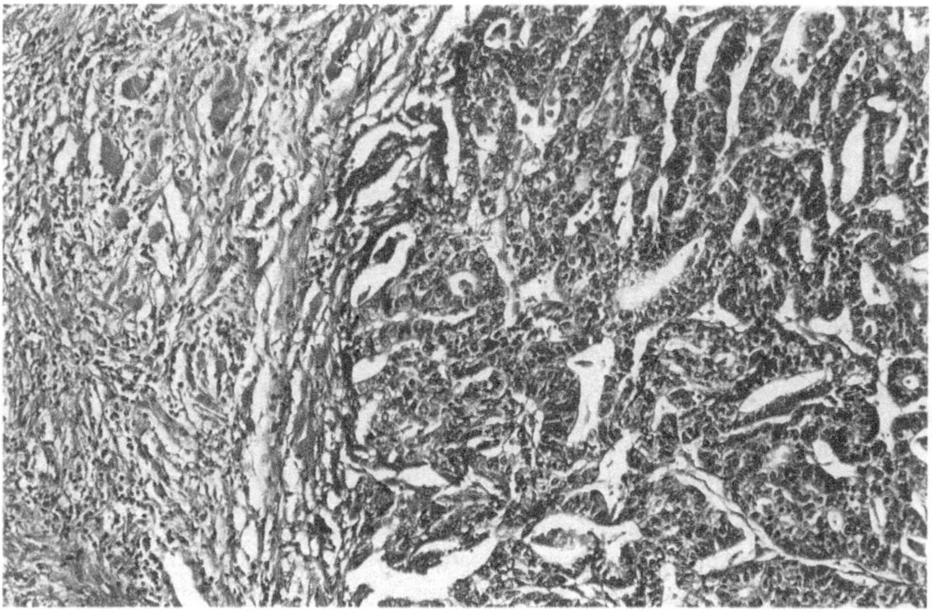

Fig. 3. Gastric carcinoma of the intestinal type (chromophotograph).

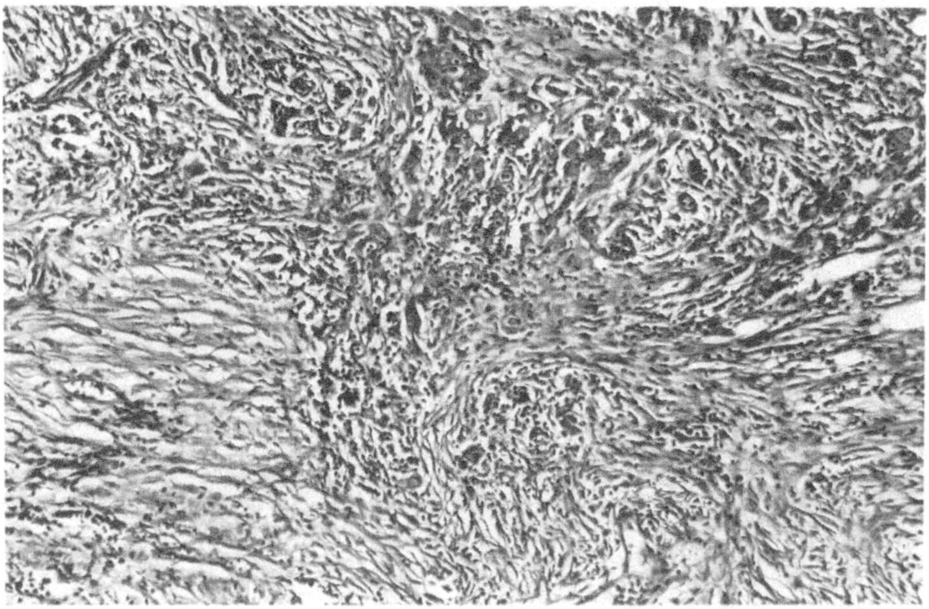

Fig. 4. Gastric carcinoma of the diffuse type (chromophotograph).

recommendations suggest that the tumor be classified according to the most unfavorable (most poorly differentiated) component.

The WHO classification is not altogether satisfactory in terms of the information it provides for prognosis. Even though a worse prognosis distinguishes the undifferentiated carcinoma from most remaining WHO types, no significant differences exist between signet-ring cell carcinoma and the various adenocarcinomas. Grading the adenocarcinomas also results in no significant prognostic information.[7,8]

Laurén Classification

The Laurén classification[9,10] distinguishes between the intestinal and diffuse types (Table 1; Figs. 3 and 4). Categorization occurs solely on the basis of histological criteria. Tumors that are nonhomogeneous with respect to Laurén are categorized by predominant type, according to the proposals of Munoz and associates.[11]

Most important from the clinical and surgical standpoints is the behavior of both Laurén types at the macroscopic edge of the tumor. While indistinguishable in the stage of early carcinoma (infiltration in mucosa or in submucosa), it most certainly may be distinguished in the more advanced tumors. In the intestinal type, growth beyond the macroscopic edge of the tumor is found only on a short segment measuring several millimeters. In contrast, the advanced diffuse type—primarily in the proximal direction—often reveals an expansion in a macroscopically normal gastric wall which may be detected only histologically, often several centimeters away from the macroscopic edge of the tumor. This spread takes the form of discontinuous islands of tumor, mostly in the submucosa and subserosa. In tumors of the upper half of the stomach, carcinoma spreads proximally to the esophagus, while extension to the duodenum remains altogether restricted, at least in the case of curatively operable patients. Hence this variable growth behavior requires different margins of clearance in the intestinal and diffuse types, with the margin being particularly important proximally.

Table 2 shows the resulting clinical consequences. We make express mention of the fact that an intraoperative frozen section examination of the oral edge of the resection is not expedient given the selection of a smaller margin of clearance. Such a section would reveal only a continuous spread of tumor up to the edge of the resection, but not the discontinuous tumor islands remaining in the gastric wall. The margins of clearance must be expanded to eliminate or remove the latter as well. The requirement for choosing different margins of clearance in accordance with the stage and Laurén type stems primarily from the differing growth behavior as revealed above all by the histological examination of large block sections. An analysis of our patients confirms these requirements. The frequency of local recurrences may be significantly reduced[12,13] and the 5-year survival rate increased significantly[14,15] by observing the appropriate margins of clearance. Even when classifying patients according to the latest UICC stages,[16,17] the long-term prognosis becomes better in a diffuse carcinoma when an oral margin of

Table 2. Margins of clearance as a function of Laurén type[a]

Necessary oral margins of clearance	In situ	On fresh resection specimen without tension
Early carcinoma	> 4–5 cm	> 2–3 cm
Advanced carcinoma, Intestinal type	> 4–5 cm	> 2–3 cm
Advanced carcinoma, Diffuse type	> 8–10 cm	> 4–5 cm

[a]These values vary greatly depending on the measuring condition.

Planning of surgery	
1. Early gastric cancer (every type) and advanced intestinal carcinoma	
Localization in upper half	Total gastrectomy; abdominal in general, abdominothoracic when extending to esophagus
Localization in lower half	Subtotal distal gastrectomy
2. Advanced carcinoma, diffuse type	
In general total gastrectomy	
Localization in lower third of stomach	Abdominal
Localization in middle and/or upper third of stomach	Abdominothoracic (with appropriately wide resection of thoracic esophagus)
In the case of small prepyloric tumors subtotal distal gastrectomy possible	

clearance in excess of 5 cm (measured on the fresh resection specimen without tension) is observed (Table 3).

Prognosis

Tumor Removal (Resectability)

Prognosis following a diagnosis of gastric cancer depends primarily on whether the tumor can be surgically removed (Table 4A). The 5-year survival rate in

Table 3. Prognosis following curative removal of diffuse type carcinomas[a]

Stages	Oral margin of clearance (cm)	n	5-Year survival rates with 95% confidence limit	Median survival time (mo)	Statistical significance of differences (P)
II	≤ 5	32	40 ± 24%	31.7	ns
	> 5	18	60 ± 40%	59.4	
III	≤ 5	58	7 ± 11%	13.2	<.01
	> 5	32	50 ± 23%	21.7	

[a]Dependence on proximal margin of clearance (measured on the fresh resection specimen without tension). 5-Year survival rates (according to actuarial method, age-corrected) and median survival time. Postoperative deaths not included. Surgical University Clinic, Erlangen, June 15 1977–December 31 1984/December 31 1986.

Table 4. Prognosis as a function of resectability and R classification[a]

Patient groups	n	5-Year survival rates with 95% confidence limits	Median survival (mo)	Statistically significant differences (*P*)
A. Resectability				
All patients	905	32 ± 4%	12.7	
Tumor not removed	244	0%	3.1	.01
Tumor removed	661	44 ± 5%	24.9	
B. R Classification				
R0	519	54 ± 6%	42.1	R0/R1 and R0/R2: < .01
R1	39	8 ± 10%	13.1	
R2	103	5 ± 5%	6.8	R1/R2: ns
R1,2	142	6 ± 5%	7.7	

[a] 5-Year survival rates (according to the actuarial method, age-corrected) and median survival time. Postoperative deaths not included. Surgical University Clinic, Erlangen, June 15 1977–December 31 1984/December 31 1986.

patients whose tumor was not removed was 0%, in contrast to a 5-year survival rate of 44% in patients whose tumor was resected. Median survival times are correspondingly different (3.1 vs. 24.9 months).

R Classification

Extremely important prognostic differences according to the R classification first result within the group of patients who underwent tumor resection (Table 4B). A distinction is drawn between R0, no residual tumor; R1, microscopic residual tumor; and R2, macroscopic residual tumor.[16,17]

R0 corresponds to the potentially curative resection. Only with the latter can satisfactory results be expected, while the prognosis is very unfavorable given a residual tumor.

pTNM Classification

The group of tumors that might potentially be removed curatively (R0) is not at all homogeneous, with the 5-year survival rates ranging from 90% to 0%. This is why another classification must be adopted for R0 patients. As shown in Table 5, the stage grouping of the UICC, valid effective 1987, has been proven effective for these cases. A very clear and highly significant dependence of prognosis on stage is demonstrated in this case (Table 6).

Other Prognostic Factors

The current stage grouping of the UICC takes into account only the anatomic spread of the tumor. However, other parameters are involved in a prognosis

Table 5. pTNM Classification and stage grouping of UICC[a]

TNM Clinical Classification

T = Primary tumor

TX	Primary tumor cannot be assessed
T0	No evidence of primary tumor
Tis	Carcinoma in situ: intraepithelial tumor without invasion of the lamina propria
T1	Tumor invades lamina propria or submucosa
T2	Tumor invades muscularis propria or subserosa[1]
T3	Tumor penetrates the serosa (visceral peritoneum) without invasion of adjacent structures[2,3]
T4	Tumor invades adjacent structures[2,3]

Notes: (1) A tumor may penetrate muscularis propria with extension into the gastrocolic or gastrohepatic ligaments or the greater or lesser omentum without perforation of the visceral peritoneum covering these structures. In this case, the tumor is classified T2. If there is perforation of the visceral peritoneum covering the gastric ligaments or omenta, the tumor is classified T3.

(2) The adjacent structures of the stomach are the spleen, transverse colon, liver, diaphragm, pancreas, abdominal wall, adrenal gland, kidney, small intestine, and retroperitoneum.

(3) Intramural extension into the duodenum or esophagus is classified by the depth of greatest invasion in any of these sites including the stomach.

N = Regional Lymph Nodes

The regional lymph nodes are the perigastric nodes along the lesser and greater curvatures and the nodes located along the left gastric, common hepatic, splenic, and çeliac arteries. Involvement of other intraabdominal lymph nodes such as the hepatoduodenal, retropancreatic, mesenteric, and para-aortic is classified as distant metastasis.

NX	Regional lymph nodes cannot be assessed
N0	No regional lymph node metastasis
N1	Metastasis in perigastric lymph node(s) within 3 cm of the edge of the primary tumor
N2	Metastasis in perigastric lymph node(s) more than 3 cm from the edge of the primary tumor or in lymph nodes along the left gastric, common hepatic, splenic, or celiac arteries

M = Distant Metastases

MX	Presence of distant metastasis cannot be assessed
M0	No distant metastasis
M1	Distant metastasis

pTNM Pathological Classification

The pT, pN, and pM categories correspond to the T, N, and M categories.

	Stage grouping		
Stage 0	Tis	N0	M0
Stage 1A	T1	N0	M0
Stage 1B	T1	N1	M0
	T2	N0	M0
Stage II	T1	N2	M0
	T2	N1	M0
	T3	N0	M0
Stage IIIA	T2	N2	M0
	T3	N1	M0
	T4	N0	M0

	Stage grouping		
Stage IIIB	T3	N2	M0
	T4	N1	M0
Stage IV	T4	N2	M0
	Any T	Any N	M1

[a]Reproduced with permission from Hermanek P, Sobin LH (eds): UICC: TNM Classification of Malignant Tumours, ed 4. Berlin-Heidelberg-New York, Springer, 1987, p 43.

following curative tumor removal. These may be attributed to the tumor itself (in particular localization in the organ and histomorphology) or to the patients (age, sex, comorbidity, etc.). The treatment procedure must also always be taken into account.

When analyzing these many possible prognostic factors, the numerous correlations and interactions between the various factors which might simulate influences on the prognoses that may in fact not exist must be borne in mind. These intricate correlations may only be clarified by means of multivariate statistical methods, in particular the Cox model and logistic regression analysis with the simulation of nonproportional hazards.[18,19]

Such a pilot study was initiated on a strictly selected and hence homogeneous group of patients.[20] Table 7 shows the design of this study. The objective within each UICC stage was to elicit additional independent prognostic factors with a 5-year survival rate as the target parameter. The following were determined:

Stage I: Comorbidity
  Localization (lower or middle third more favorable)
Stage IIIA: Planned margin of clearance
  Number of lymph nodes involved (up to 3/over 3)
Stage IIIB: Sex (female more favorable)
  Number of involved lymph nodes

Large groups of patients are required in analyses such as these so that those factors that have a significant but not very great independent effect on the prognosis

Table 6. Prognosis after curative tumor removal (R0)[a]

Stages	n	5-Year survival rate with 95% confidence limits	Median survival time (mo)
IA	85	85 ± 14%	Undefined
IB	104	89 ± 12%	Undefined
II	114	47 ± 14%	40.9
IIIA	99	34 ± 14%	20.1
IIIB	69	21 ± 13%	13.8
IV	24	0%	10.0

[a]Dependence on UICC stage. 5-Year survival rates (according to the actuarial method, age-corrected) and median survival time. Postoperative deaths not included. Surgical University Clinic, Erlangen, June 15 1977–December 31 1984/December 31 1986.

Table 7. Multivariate analysis of prognostic factors after curative operations for gastric cancer

Patient selection:	First time with disease
(n = 533)	No previous gastric resection
	Adenocarcinoma, signet-ring cell carcinoma or undifferentiated carcinoma
	Treatment via total or subtotal distal gastrectomy
	Curative operation (R0)
	No postoperative exitus
Analyzed factors:	
Patient-related	Sex
	Age
	Comorbidity
Tumor-related:	Preoperative complications
	Localization
	Size of tumor
	Histological type according to WHO
	Degree of differentiation according to WHO
	Laurén type
	Number of involved lymph nodes
Therapy-associated:	Year of operation
	Planned proximal margin of clearance[a]
	Total v subtotal distal gastrectomy
	Splenectomy
	Additional resection of neighboring organs
	Extent of lymph-node dissection

[a] Definitions, see Table 2.

From a pilot study by Hermanek P, Guggenmoos-Holzmann I: Multivariate analysis of prognosis following curative tumor resection of stomach carcinoma, abstract from the *Proceedings of the 4th European Conference on Clinical Oncology and Cancer Nursing (ECCO)*, held at Madrid, November 1–4 1987. Madrid, Fundación para la Investigación y la Formación en Oncologia, 1987, p 32.

may be recognized. Plans are currently underway within the UICC to carry out such examinations on larger groups of patients on a multicentric and international basis. The additional prognostic factors important for each stage are to be ascertained in this way. The final aim is to expand the current stages, which took into consideration only the anatomic spread, to prognostic groups by incorporating additional independent prognostic factors including therapy. This will enable a more precise evaluation of course and a more accurate estimation of prognoses as well as establish the essential preconditions for the evaluation of therapeutic procedures and for the very important area of precisely defining indications for adjuvant chemotherapy.

References

1. Hermanek P: Dysplasia in the gastrointestinal tract: definition and clinical significance. Surg Endosc 1987;1:5.
2. Heilmann KL: Gastritis-intestinale Metaplasie – Karzinom. Stuttgart, Georg Thieme, 1978.

3. Jass JR: A classification of gastric dysplasia. Histopathology 1983;7:181.
4. Segura DI, Montero C: Histochemical characterization of different types of intestinal metaplasia in gastric mucosa. Cancer 1983;52:498.
5. Morson BC, Jass JR, Sobin LH: Precancerous Lesions of the Gastrointestinal Tract. A Histological Classification. London, Bailliere Tindall, 1985, p 5.
6. Oota K, Sobin LH: Histological typing of gastric and oesophageal tumours. International Histological Classification of Tumours. No. 18. Geneva, WHO, 1977, p 38.
7. Hermanek P: Magenkarzinom–Typing, grading, staging, in Gall FP, Hermanek P, Hornig D (eds): Magenkarzinom: Epidemiologie, Pathologie, Therapie, Nachsorge. Munich-Bern-Vienna, W Zuckschwerdt, 1986, p 36.
8. Craven J: Prognostic indices in stomach cancer, in Stoll BA (ed): Pointers to Cancer Prognosis. Dordrecht, Martinus Nijhoff, 1987, p 322.
9. Laurén P: The two histological main types of gastric carcinoma: diffuse and so-called intestinal-type carcinoma. Acta Path Microbiol Scand 1965;64:31.
10. Giedl J: Klinische Bedeutung der histologischen Typenbestimmung beim Magenkrebs. Mün Med Wschr 1980;122:205.
11. Munoz N, Correa P, Cuello C, et al: Histologic types of gastric carcinoma in high- and low-risk areas. Inter J Cancer 1968;3:809.
12. Husemann B. Altendorf A: Magenkarzinomrezidiv–eine vermeidbare Komplikation? in Jakesz R (ed): Derzeitiger Stand in Diagnose und Therapie des Magenkarzinoms. Vienna, Facultas, 1987, p 134.
13. Husemann B, Altendorf-Hofmann A: Hat der histologische Typ nach Laurén für die Planung des operativen Vorgehens bei kurativer Therapie des Magenkarzinoms Bedeutung? Langenbecks Arch Chir 1987;372:867.
14. Hermanek P, Gall FP: Intestinal and diffuse type of gastric carcinoma. Two clinical entities. J Cancer Res Clin Oncol 1986;111(suppl):82.
15. Hornig D, Hermanek P, Gall FP: The significance of the extent of proximal margin of clearance in gastric cancer surgery. Scand J Gastroenterol 1987;22(suppl 133):69.
16. Hermanek P, Sobin LH (eds): UICC: TNM Classification of Malignant Tumours, ed 4. Berlin-Heidelberg-New York, Springer, 1987, p 43.
17. Hermanek P, Scheibe O, Spiessl B, et al (eds): UICC: TNM-Klassifikation maligner Tumoren, ed 4. Berlin-Heidelberg-New York, Springer, 1987, p 45.
18. Guggenmoos-Holzmann I, Hermanek P: Multivariate Analyse der Therapieergebnisse bei kolorektalen Karzinomen, in Hermanek P (ed): Bedeutung des TNM-Systems für die klinische Onkologie. Munich-Bern-Vienna, W. Zuckschwerdt, 1986, p 223.
19. Hermanek P: Klinische Krebsforschung, in Gall FP, Hermanek P, Tonak J (eds): Chirurgische Onkologie, Histologie-und stadien-gerecht Therapie maligner Tumoren. Berlin-Heidelberg-New York, Springer, 1986, p 236.
20. Hermanek P, Guggenmoos-Holzmann I: Multivariate analysis of prognosis following curative tumor resection of stomach carcinoma, abstract from the Proceedings of the 4th European Conference on Clinical Oncology and Cancer Nursing (ECCO), held at Madrid, November 1–4 1987. Madrid, Fundación para la Investigación y la Formación en Oncologia, 1987, p 32.

Part II
Diagnosis

CHAPTER 3

Endoscopic Criteria for Premalignant Lesions and Early Gastric Carcinoma

W. Rösch

Introduction

Since the introduction of fiber endoscopy in the late 1960s, a fundamental change—which cannot be underestimated—has occurred in the diagnosis of gastric carcinoma. Fewer than 3% of all cancers diagnosed in the preendoscopic era were in the early stages, but with the advent of endoscopy this figure has already reached 15% to 20% at some centers and has surpassed 60% in Japan, where endoscopic screening programs were established early on.

Following a suggestion by Heinkel and associates,[1] the quality of an endoscopy department is currently judged by the number of diagnoses of early gastric carcinoma, which should total at least 10% of all diagnosed cancers. Despite many critical objections, the classification of early gastric carcinoma adopted in 1962 by the Japan Gastrointestinal Endoscopic Society and in 1963 by the Japanese Cancer Research Society has gained worldwide acceptance (Fig. 1), with early gastric carcinoma present in cases where the cancer growth is limited to the surface layer, ie, the mucosa or mucosa and submucosa. Otherwise viewed as a criterion of advanced carcinoma, lymph-node metastases are not considered.

The special position occupied by early gastric carcinoma is justified by the excellent prognosis of this disease. Takasugi and associates[2] reported a 100% survival rate in 724 cases of early mucosal carcinoma, and a 95% survival rate in cases of infiltration of the submucosa.

Endoscopic diagnosis permits the tentative diagnosis of early carcinoma only when a relatively small lesion is apparently involved. Suspected cases are confirmed in the resection specimen, with "downstaging" being necessary roughly 20% of the time. Nonetheless, suspicion of early carcinoma based on the classic endoscopic point of view will be addressed subsequently, since the surgical procedure and particularly subtle histological workups depend on it (Fig. 2).

Endoscopic Description of Tumor Types

Early carcinomas can be diagnosed only when one is familiar with their macroscopic appearance. In addition to the types shown in Fig. 1, combined forms, such as type IIa + IIc, also occur. The latter involve a flat prominent lesion with

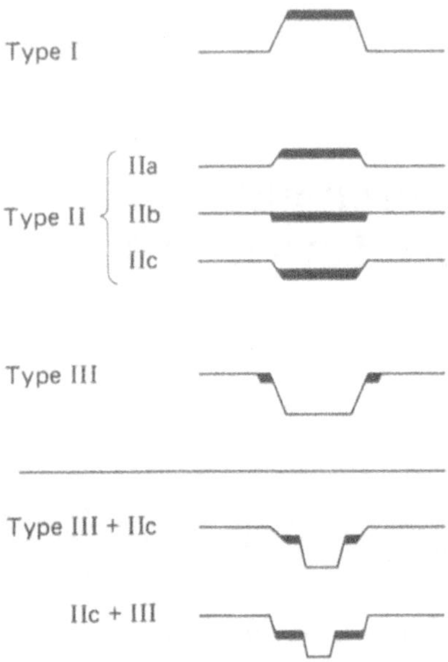

Fig. 1. Classification of early gastric cancers.

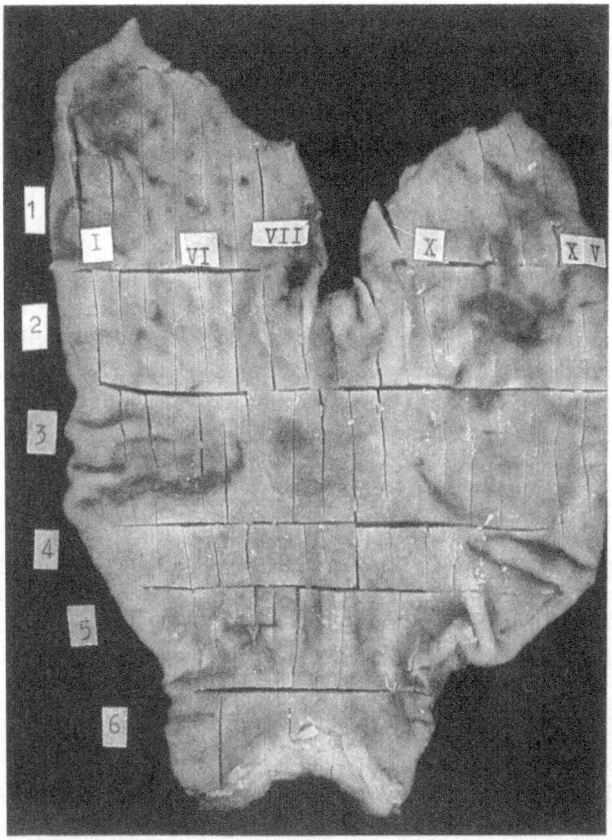

Fig. 2. Histological workup of an early gastric carcinoma.

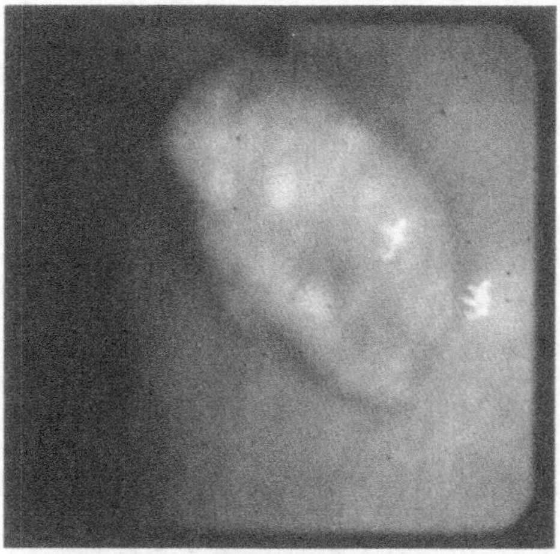

Fig. 3. Early carcinoma, type I.

a slight central depression, with the dominating portion named first. Polypoid types of early gastric carcinoma (type I) protrude at least 5 mm over the surface of the mucous membrane, with no limitation on size (Fig. 3). Precancerous structures may often still be detected in the tumor, with a highly differentiated adenocarcinoma being present from a histological standpoint.

Pronounced atrophic gastritis with intestinal metaplasia is almost always on hand in the tumor environment. Type IIa early gastric carcinoma protrudes a maximum of 5 mm over the level of the mucosa (Fig. 4). A well-differentiated adenocarcinoma is involved as well. While the type I carcinoma probably develops from a tubular adenoma, a flat adenoma (borderline lesion, protruded type) is more than likely the matrix for the type IIa cancer.

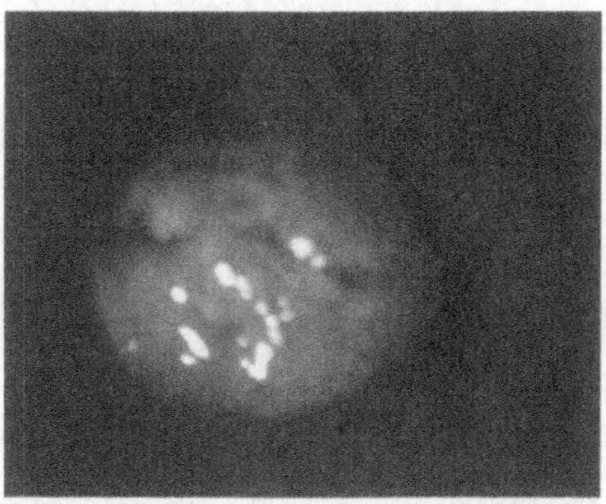

Fig. 4. Early gastric carcinoma, type IIa.

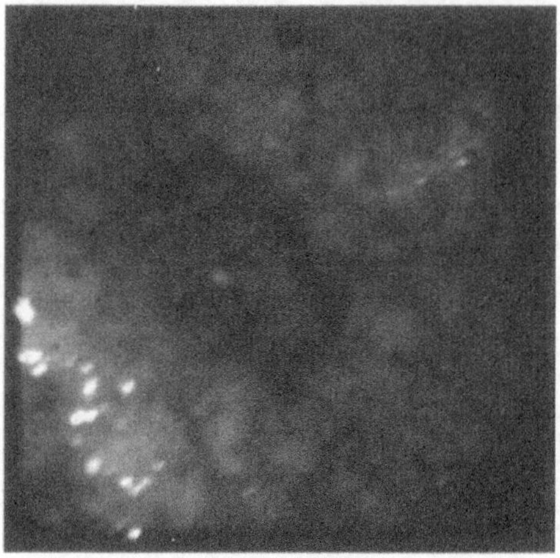

Fig. 5. Early gastric carcinoma, type IIb.

Type IIb carcinoma is normally a pure mucosal carcinoma, with infiltration of the submucosa being extremely rare.[3] Diagnosis is difficult, since the growth of the cancer might be identified only by a discoloration of the mucosa (Fig. 5). Generally a signet-ring cell carcinoma, often covered by a normal mucosa, is involved in these cases.[4] Type IIc carcinoma is the most frequent kind of early gastric carcinoma and is a flat, depressed, sometimes quite extensive lesion with central ulceration (Fig. 6). The macroscopic aspect—especially the fold configuration (Fig. 7)—is so distinctive that problems of differential diagnosis are encountered only rarely. Classically, a mucus-forming adenocarcinoma is involved, with often indistinct tumor boundaries.

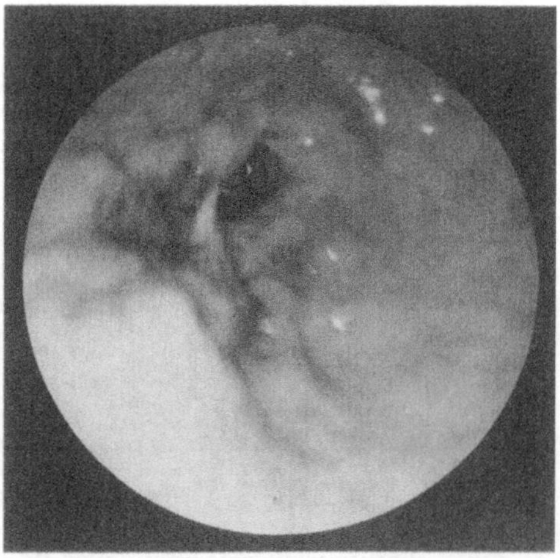

Fig. 6. Early gastric carcinoma, type IIc.

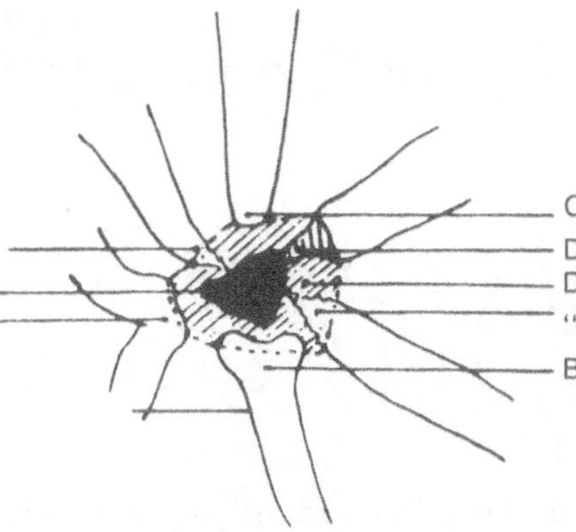

Fig. 7. Fold configuration in a malignant ulcer.

Type III is a so-called malignant ulcer, with the cancer growth extending primarily to the edge of the tumor. Partial peptic digestion of a superficial carcinoma or a benign ulcer in a malignantly transformed mucosa is involved (Fig. 8). Frequently present, however, are mixtures of IIc and III tumors, which go through a malignant cycle[5] that may go as far as an ulcer scar with consecutive relapse. The Laurén classification is vital for further procedure, in particular the prognostic assessment: types I and IIa are almost exclusively carcinomas of intestinal cells,[6] with diffuse carcinoma predominating in types IIb, IIc and III. Representative biopsy samples may only be obtained using a standardized procedure (Fig. 9). While diagnostic polypectomies were still required several years ago, the forceps biopsy is currently in use again, since it provides a sufficient level of diagnostic reliability, given an experienced pathologist. Dye procedures

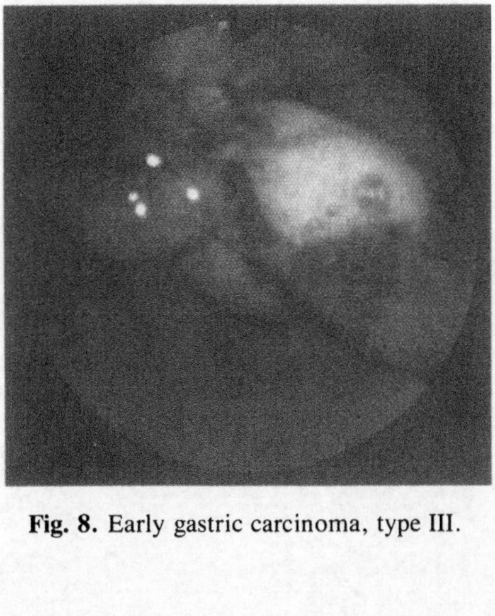

Fig. 8. Early gastric carcinoma, type III.

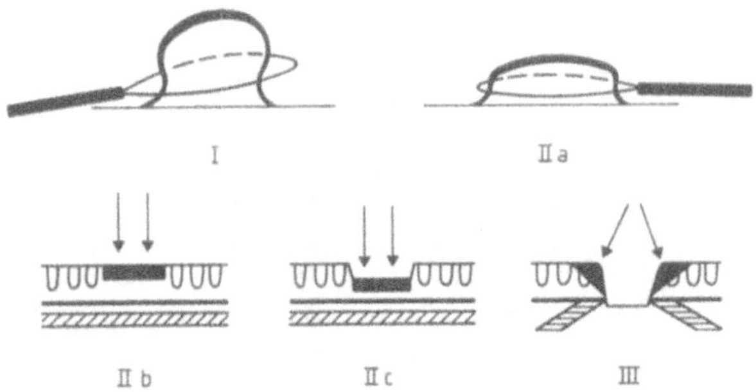

Fig. 9. Standardized procedure in suspected early gastric cancer.

(dye scattering, intravital staining) for identifying small mucosal cancers have been unable to gain acceptance. While suspected lesions may be visualized better by spraying on dyes, defining the tumor boundaries more precisely is not possible, since diffuse carcinomas in particular often undergo discontinuous, indeterminate growth.[7] Even intravital staining with methylene blue did not live up to expectations, since only 46% of the earlier cancers could be stained with this substance according to studies conducted by Hashimoto and associates.[8] The differentiation of intestinal metaplasia using alcian blue PAS dye in acid and neutral sulfated mucin for purposes of identifying intestinal metaplasia of the colon[9] is preferably practiced with resection preparations.

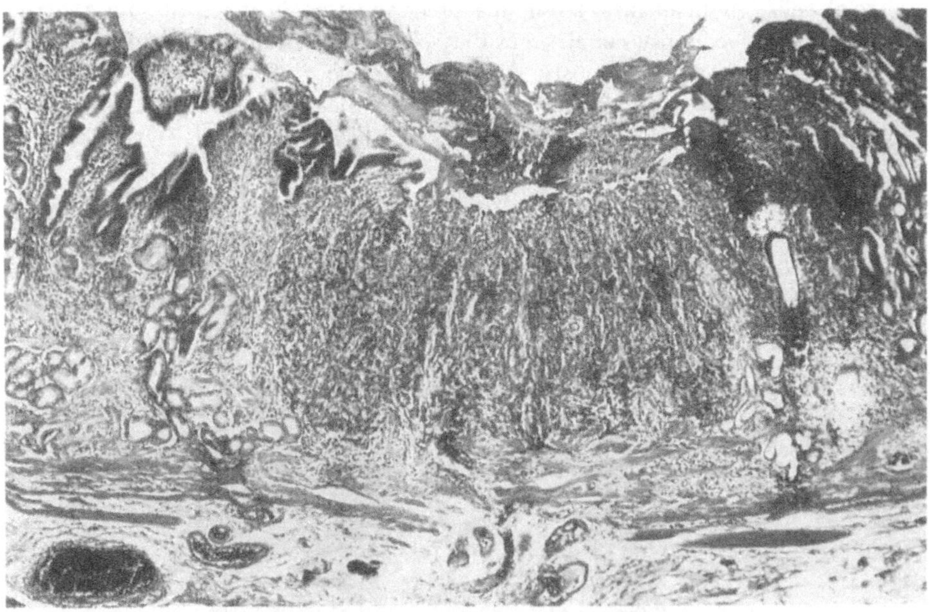

Fig. 10. Early gastric carcinoma 1 × 2 mm in diameter, impressive as erosion.

Clinical Findings

The association between benign and malignant lesions has been pointed out repeatedly. Neeman and associates[10] emphasized the association of early gastric carcinoma with duodenal ulcers, while Biasco and associates[11] (1987) found gastric polyps in 22 of 80 patients with early carcinoma, 16 of which were hyperplastic. The multicentric growth of early cancers has been alluded to frequently as well,[12] with figures of around 10% corresponding to our own experience.

Gastroscopic examination of a symptomatic patient (only 6% to 8% of all early gastric carcinomas proceed asymptomatically) includes a careful inspection of the entire stomach, with a biopsy of all circumscribed mucosal findings according to a standardized procedure. This is especially true for all gastric ulcers, in which six to eight tissue samples are to be taken from the edge of the ulcer and one or two from its base. The biopsy is worthwhile even in the case of tiny, solitary fibrin-covered lesions (Fig. 10), since exudation of fibrin is an early indication of an abnormal mucosa. Chronic, multiple erosions are almost always an exception.

The situation is more difficult in the inevitable precancerous stages of the gastric mucosa.[13] On the one hand, no uniform nomenclature exists (Table 1), while on the other, the term "dysplasia," which contains a macroscopically recognizable correlate only in part, comes into consideration (Table 2). The tendency today is to distinguish tubular adenoma (Table 3) from flat adenoma, with the former lesion corresponding to adenoma of the colon (Fig. 11) and the flat adenoma only revealing cellular atypia in the mucosa close to the surface.

The macroscopic aspect of this change, rarely exceeding 2 cm in diameter and preferably localized in the antrum, is quite typical (Fig. 12). Observations on the course of this disease in Japan show that these lesions may develop into a carcinoma, but also into the ripened form of an intestinal metaplasia. Attempts will be made to remove the inevitable precancerous stages with the diathermic loop or

Table 1. Terminology of Gastric Polyps

1. Non-neoplastic epithelial polyps
Hyperplastic (Elster)
Regenerative (Morson)
Hyperplastic (Ming)
2. Neoplastic polyps
Adenoma
Highly differentiated
Moderately differentiated
Borderline lesion, protruded type (Nagayo)
Flat adenoma (Ming)
Type III polyp (Nakamura)
Subtype Ia (Fukuchi)

Table 2A. Classification of gastric mucosa dysplasias

Nagayo Group	1 Normal	2 Slightly Atypical	3 Borderline Lesion	4 Probable Carcinoma	5 Definite Carcinoma
Ming	1 Regenerative changes	2 Proliferative changes	3 Dysplasia	4 Borderline	
WHO group	Regenerative changes	Slight	← Dysplasia →	Severe	
ISGGC	Simple hyperplasia	Atypical hyperplasia	Dysplasia	Borderline lesion	

ISGGC, International Study Group for Gastric Cancer.

Table 2B. ISGGC nomenclature of gastric dysplasias

Characteristic	Simple Hyperplasia	Atypical Hyperplasia	Dysplasia	Borderline Lesion
Cystic dilation	++	++	+	+
Glandular branching	++	++	+	+
Mucous	+++	++	±	+
N/C ratio			↑	↑
Shape of nucleus	Normal	Normal	Rod-shaped	Rod-shaped
Nucleus localization	Basal	Basal	Central/surface	Central/surface
Pseudostratification	±	+	+++	+++
Mitoses	±	+	++	+++

to resect the latter (local excision or resection of part of the stomach) despite the admittedly low associated malignancy rate. Even laser therapy appears possible in cases of flat adenoma. Patients who developed such a precancerous lesion in the stomach require gastroscopic follow-ups, especially since the association with early cancer or multicentric growth is not a rarity.[7] Follow-up examinations at 6- to 12-month intervals following endoscopic resection are apparently sufficient for detecting relapses. Endoscopic therapy of early gastric carcinoma is

Table 3. Macroscopic aspect of hyperplastic polyps and adenoma

Characteristic	Hyperplastic Polyp	Adenoma
Multiplicity	Frequent	Occasional
Localization	Entire stomach	Antrum, cardia
Average size	1 cm	4 cm
Shape	Round or oval	Papillary or villous
Contour	Smooth	Irregular
Indentation	Missing	Present
Base	Sharply delineated	Flowing
Peduncle	Thin	Broad-based

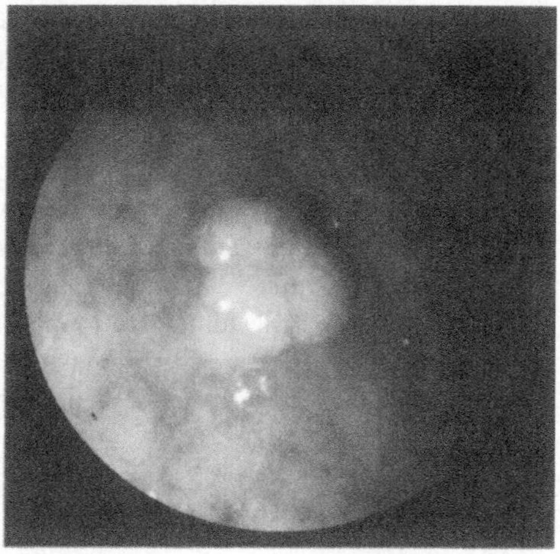

Fig. 11. Adenoma of the gastric mucosa.

permitted only in exceptional cases, and not even the recently publicized laser therapy is without its problems.[14] In our experience, the local resection of early gastric carcinoma undergoing polypoid growth is an option, given the following:

- mucosal carcinoma
- high-risk surgery
- localization in the upper third of the stomach
- high degree of differentiation
- guaranteed routine follow-up examinations.

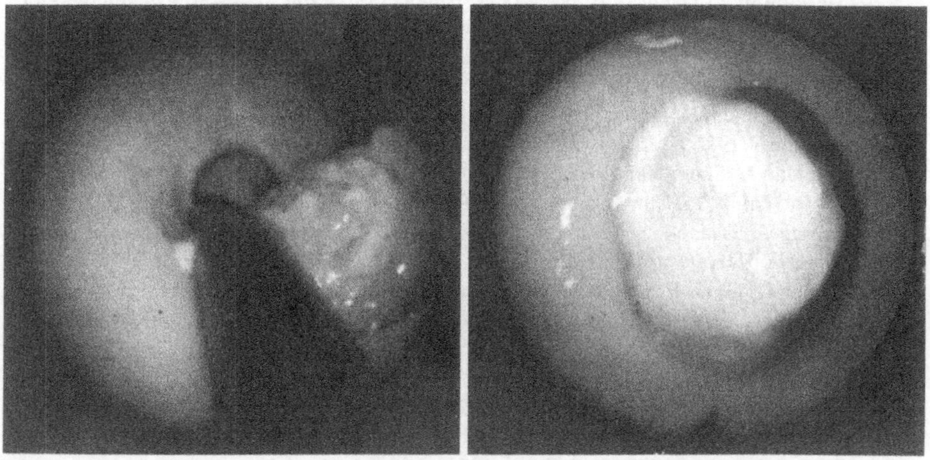

Fig. 12. Borderline lesion, protruded type (flat adenoma).

The main precondition is that the cancer be successfully removed in the healthy individual. One must even then reckon with the possibility that metastasis to the regional lymph nodes has already occurred in 2% to 3% of the cases. Gastric carcinoma may be easily detected early via endoscopic examination techniques. Why gastric anamnesis of a patient having early cancer often goes on for a considerably longer period of time than the symptoms in a patient with advanced carcinoma remains unclear. Apparently, surface growth is slow and deep infiltration rapid.[15] Kawai and associates[16] have calculated that it takes 577 to 3,462 days for the tumor to double in the case of early gastric carcinoma. While this provides time for diagnosis, it should not be taken up by systematic therapy, but rather by controlled endoscopic diagnosis.

References

1. Heinkel K, Kimmig JM, v Gaisberg U, et al: Das Magenfrühkarzinom (Eigene Statistik). Akt Gastrol 1976;5:227.
2. Takasugi T, Hirota T, Sasagawa M: Actuarial survival rate of early gastric cancer. Stomach Intestine 1977;12:933.
3. Fernando SSE, Nakamura K: Japanese technique of early gastric cancer diagnosis. Am J Gastroenterol 1986;81:757.
4. Yamashina M: A variant of early gastric carcinoma. Histologic and histochemical studies of early signet ring cell carcinomas discovered beneath preserved surface epithelium. Cancer 1986;58:1333.
5. Sakita T, Oguro Y, Takasu S, et al: Observations on the healing of ulceration in early gastric cancer. Gastroenterology 1971;60:835.
6. Elster K, Seifert E: Magenfrühkarzinom. Baden-Baden, Witzstrock, 1979.
7. Rösch W, Frühmorgen P: Endoscopic treatment of precanceroses and early gastric carcinoma. Endoscopy 1980;12:109.
8. Hashimoto Y, Takada S, Kohli Y, et al: Application of blue dye scattering method for recognizing early gastric cancer. Proc 2nd Asian Pacific Congress of Endoscopy, 1976, p 202.
9. Turani H, Lurie B, Chaimoff C, et al: The diagnostic significance of sulfated acid mucin content in gastric intestinal metaplasia with early gastric cancer. Am J Gastroenterol 1986;81:343.
10. Neeman A, Shoenfeld Y, Kadish U: Does duodenal ulcer lead to an early diagnosis of gastric cancer? J Clin Gastroenterol 1987;9:37.
11. Biasco G, Paganelli GM, Azzaroni D: Early gastric cancer in Italy. Clinical and pathological observations of 80 cases. Dig Dis Sci 1987;32:113.
12. Miller G, Gloor F: Das Magenfrühkarzinom. Schweiz Med Wschr 1986;116:1366.
13. Rösch W, Elster K: Gastrointestinale Präkanzerosen. Baden-Baden, Witzstrock, 1977.
14. Tajiri H, Daikuzono N, Joffe SN, et al: Photoradiation therapy in early gastrointestinal cancer. Gastrointest Endosc 1987;33:88.
15. Fujita S, Ashihara T: Growth and proliferation, in Sugano H, Kobayashi J (eds): Tumor Pathology. Tokyo, Asakura, 1970, p 39.
16. Kawai K, Miyaoka T, Kohli Y: Evaluation of early gastric cancer from the clinical point of view, in Grundmann E, Grunze H, Witte S (eds): Early Gastric Cancer: Current Status of Diagnosis. Berlin-Heidelberg-New York, Springer, 1974, p 63.

CHAPTER 4

Clinical Staging of Gastric Cancer by Ultrasound, Computerized Tomography, and Magnetic Resonance Tomography

R. Grote, H.-J. Meyer, H. Milbradt,
J. Jähne, and P. Heintz

Introduction

The stage of a malignant disease is determined by the primary tumor as well as by the presence or absence of lymph nodes or organ metastases. The diagnostic procedures usually employed in the primary diagnosis of malignant gastric disease – endoscopy and X-ray double-contrast examinations – only determine the endoluminary spread and hence only part of the primary tumor.

Imaging procedures – sonography, computerized tomography, and, most recently, magnetic resonance tomography (MR) – can provide additional information about involvement of parenchymal organs or lymph nodes. The question arises of whether a reliable stage classification of malignant tumors is possible by means of these imaging procedures. Endoscopic sonography, which is currently in a clinically experimental stage, will not be considered in this discussion.

Our experience is based on a prospective series of 64 CT scans which we conducted from 1983 to 1984 in patients with malignant growths.[1] In order to ascertain the various tumor stages we attempted to examine all patients with suspected gastric neoplasia (59 carcinomas, 3 non-Hodgkin's lymphomas, 2 chronic gastric ulcers) waiting for surgery at the Medical University of Hannover, Federal Republic of Germany. More than 200 CT scans involving the identically formulated problem were prepared in a routine program in the period that followed, with a relatively large proportion of cardiac tumors.

Preoperative sonography was carried out from 1986 to 1987 on 97 patients. Thirty-nine of these were specially prepared and their stomachs were filled with water. We employed the 1978 version of the TNM classification to evaluate the sonograms as well as the CT scans.

Studies on the use of sonography or CT during gastric diseases have appeared over the last 10 years.[1,2–13] Because these publications use different tumor classifications or lack comparisons with the surgical findings, only a few of the more recent studies can be considered.[1,4,5,7,10,11] Concerning MR tomography, there are only a few publications about its application in gastric tumors. To date we have examined three cases.

Preparation

The application of imaging procedures in gastric diagnosis requires special preparation. The stomach must be empty to prevent a false interpretation caused by food particles. A 4-hour period of fasting before the procedure usually suffices, although this must be extended in the case of pyloric stenosis. Since the thickness of the gastric wall depends on the condition of fullness, and the folds of the gastric wall may mimic a tumor, our aim is to distend the stomach completely.

Immediately prior to sonography, the patient receives 800 to 1,000 ml of fruit juice or plain tap water to which polydimethyl siloxane has been added to remove foam from the stomach (Sab simplex®, Ceolate®). To delay evacuation of the stomach, a spasmolytic (eg, 40 mg butylscopolamine [Buscopan®], 1 mg glucagon) is also injected.

In preparation for CT scanning we administer 700 ml of a 2.75–3% Gastrographin solution following the injection of Buscopan® or glucagon to reduce peristaltically induced artifacts. The patient lying in the device is allowed to drink another 100 ml through a straw in order to contrast the esophagus. Filling with liquid, currently water, and medicinal relaxation precede MR tomography as well.

Primary Tumor

Sonographically, the normal gastric wall comprises five layers. In the CT scan the well distended gastric wall normally shows up as a narrow strip which may appear somewhat more widened near the cardia and in the antrum.[8] Pathological changes on the sonogram manifest themselves as a thickening of the gastric wall, typically as a circular expansion recalling a "target" pattern. Discrete pathological changes point to a disruption in the layer structure, so that early carcinomas may be discovered. A change in the wall could be detected in 67% of cases in which the stomach was unfilled and in 85% of those in which it was filled with water. Tumors of the corpus and antrum region were easier to diagnose than were those in the region of the cardia and fundus.

As a rule, depth of infiltration could not be determined reliably. According to the literature, tumors could be detected in 87 to 95% of cases, while the depth of infiltration in cases of growth exceeding the organ was assessed correctly in 75 to 85%.[1,4] One explanation for our relatively unfavorable results may be the relatively large number of proximal carcinomas.

In our prospective series of 64 patients the CT scan showed 95% of tumors as circumscribed or as diffuse wall thickening. No correlate was found in only two of six T1 tumors. The results of our remaining examinations were in the same range, with advanced tumor stages predominant in this group, but with a larger share of proximal malignant growth as well. Published data indicate a detection accuracy of approximately 90%.[2,3,5,10,11] In agreement with other investigators, we were unable to differentiate among tumors of the T1, T2, and T3 stages. Initially we believed that an indistinct tumor boundary with fine branches into the surrounding fatty tissue might provide a criterion for a T3 stage, but similar changes could be detected in 44% of T2 tumors as well.

Direct contact between the tumor and adjacent organs or an infiltration of the separating fatty layer alone is not sufficient for diagnosis of a T4 stage. Changes in shape or structure must also be evident. Special problems arise in slender or cachectic patients, in whom the fatty layer, particularly between the stomach and pancreas, is already eliminated. In these cases a change in position with the detection of a displacement between the tumor and adjacent organs may be of benefit.

The correct classification was made in 84% of the cases in our prospective series. A pancreatic infiltration which could not be confirmed histologically was assumed in two (15%) of 13 cases. In these patients, adhesions between the stomach and pancreas were found at surgery. Figures of 54% to 90% correct T4 classifications have been reported, with both false-positive and false-negative assessments.[3,4,9,10,11]

The MR tomogram shows a thickening of the gastric wall corresponding to the CT scan.

In terms of differential diagnosis, it should be noted that on ultrasound and CT an incomplete distention of the gastric wall, inflammatory disease, ulcers, or benign tumors may cause a thickening of the gastric wall resembling an infiltrating or polypous tumor growth.

Lymph Nodes

Pathologically altered lymph nodes may be detected by all three procedures at the curvatures, in the hilus of the liver and spleen, peripancreatically, in the area of the celiac artery, the mesenteric superior artery, and the para-aortic region. Para-esophageal and mediastinal lymph node metastases which occur during neoplasms near the cardia can be imaged only by CT or MR tomography.

By sonography we were able to detect lymph-node metastases correctly in liquid-filled stomachs in 69%, but only in 33% of the cases otherwise. Stages of tumor in our prospective series were exactly classified according to the TNM scheme about 80% with CT. The CT results obtained from our routine patients were worse and corresponded to those already reported with a 70 to 75% detection accuracy, as did the sonographic values.[1-7,9-14] Para-aortic lymph nodes and lymph nodes located near the celiac artery can be detected more accurately than those located at the curvatures. In CT, differentiating vessels and lymph nodes may require a bolus injection of a contrast agent. Vessels tended to be detected clearly in sonography and MR tomography.

False-negative findings in our patients were generally based on tumorous lymph nodes smaller than 5 mm, a size below the resolution of the sonographic and CT devices.

Contrary to earlier published articles by American authors,[2,9] false-positive as well as false-negative findings must also be considered. We discovered enlarged lymph nodes – twice via sonography and four times via CT – up to 20 mm in size which were confirmed surgically, but without histological sign of metastatic involvement.

Distant Metastases

In about 80% of cases sonography and CT correctly detected distant metastases in abdominal organs. Published data range between 60% and 90%.[1-14] Findings classified as false-negative in part corresponded to small superficial liver metastases. In one patient an intraparenchymal liver metastasis was not detected in the CT and also could not be recognized retrospectively.

Peritoneal carcinosis must be assumed in the presence of ascites. Linear densities in the peritoneal fatty tissue may indicate a peritoneal involvement, with the size generally being underestimated.

Summary

Sonography and CT may be helpful diagnostic tools for the staging of primary gastric malignant tumors. Detection of infiltration into neighboring organs is successful in approximately 70 to 80% of cases, with some false-positives occurring. Lymph-node metastases are correctly determined 70 to 80%, with false-positives as well as false-negatives occurring. Organ metastases are correctly recognized in 80% of cases. Detection of peritoneal carcinosis without ascites is problematic. Overall, CT is superior to sonography, with each procedure complementing the other.

MR tomography cannot yet be judged satisfactorily. With the appropriate technique, CT may be expected to yield corresponding results. The visibility of vessels by MR is beneficial. General application of CT in particular is not recommended, but seems to be useful in gastroesophageal tumors with a possible spread to the mediastinum. Exploratory laparotomies may be avoided in special cases, in which ultrasound and CT show a broad extension of the disease.

Follow-up examinations of unresectable tumors, especially during chemotherapy, represent a new indication.

References

1. Derchi LE, Biggi E, Rolandi GA, et al: Sonographic staging of gastric cancer. Am J Roentgenol 1983;140:273.
2. Freeny PC, Marks WM: Adenocarcinoma of the gastroesophageal junction: barium and CT-examination. Am J Roentgenol 1982;138:1077.

3. Grosser G, Wimmer B, Ruf G: Diagnostischer Wert der Computertomographie beim Magenkarzinom. Fortschr Roentgenstr 1985;142:514.
4. Grosser G, Brambs H-J, Wimmer B, et al: Sonographische Darstellung und Beurteilung von Magenwandveränderungen. Fortschr Roentgenstr 1987;147:79.
5. Grote R, Döhring W, Meyer H-J, et al: Computertomographie bei malignen Tumoren des Magens. Fortschr Roentgenstr 1984;141:654.
6. Komaki S: Normal or benign gastric wall thickening demonstrated by computed tomography. J Comp Assist Tomogr 1982;6:1103.
7. Milbradt H, Jähne J, Meyer H-J, et al: Die Bedeutung der Sonographie beim präoperativen Staging des Magenkarzinoms. Fortschr Roentgenstr, in press.
8. Marks WM, Callen PW, Moss AA: Gastroesophageal region: Source of confusion on CT. Am J Roentgenol 1981;136:359.
9. Moss AA, Schnyder P, Marks W, et al: Gastric adenocarcinoma: A comparison of the accuracy and economics of staging by computed tomography and surgery. Gastroenterology 1981;80:45.
10. Schröder R, Triller J, Roder R: Wert der Computertomographie beim fortgeschrittenen Magenkarzinom. Ist die Probelaparotomie vermeidbar? Schweiz medz Wschr 1986;116:956.
11. Triller J, Roder R, Stafford A, et al: CT in advanced gastric carcinoma: is exploratory laparotomy avoidable? Eur J Radiol 1986;6:181.
12. Winkler ML: MR imaging of diffusely infiltrating gastric carcinoma. J Comp Assist Tomogr 1987;11:337.
13. Worlicek H, Lederer P, Lux G: Ultrasonographic evaluation of the wall of the fluid filled stomach—case report of a leiomyoblastoma. Hepato-gastroenterol 1986; 33:184.
14. Yeh H-C, Rabinowitz JG: Ultrasonography and computed tomography of gastric wall lesions. Radiology 1981;141:147.

Part III
Surgical Therapy of Gastric Carcinoma

CHAPTER 5

Surgical Treatment of Gastric Carcinoma: Approach According to Tumor Stage or Total Gastrectomy as the Operation of Choice

H.-J. Meyer, J. Jähne, and R. Pichlmayr

Introduction

Although the incidence of gastric carcinoma is declining, epidemiologic investigations show that this tumor continues to be one of the leading causes of death from cancer.[1-5] Even with increasingly differentiated diagnostic procedures and improved standardization of histopathologic classifications, the requirements for early diagnosis and sufficient radicality as basic preconditions for therapy remain as pressing as ever, since the extent of surgery continues to be a major topic of discussion, regardless of changed points of view.

Depending on the particular opinion, this can relate to the level of radicality at the tumor-bearing organ (ie, the importance of total gastrectomy as the operation of choice compared with the stage-dependent or histologically oriented approach), as well as to the influence of therapeutic value of systematic lymphadenectomy and/or obligatory splenectomy.[1,3-30] Since only scattered, if any, valid preliminary data from controlled clinical studies are available at this time, the discussion must remain open. Nonetheless, some facts do aid in selecting a therapeutic procedure more objectively or indicate that contrary points of view have clearly been reconciled.

Current Status of the Surgical Approach

Although the indications for necessary total gastrectomy have remained unquestioned and broadly accepted for a long time, even for palliation alone,[1,3,5-7,10,14,20,23,24] controversy persists regarding the value and importance of routine gastrectomy in the early tumor stages, particularly in early gastric carcinomas.*

The original concept of total gastrectomy "de principe" was based primarily on the general confusion and difficulty concerning the level of radicality required when selecting resection lines at the stomach; in particular, the last point was of

*Refs. 1, 3, 5–8, 10, 14, 16, 18–27, 31.

Table 1. Postoperative mortality following total gastrectomy: literature review

Author	Year	Total (n)	Operative mortality (%)
Peiper	1978[a]	2,726	23.7
Hollender	1982[a]	1,355	18.0
Re Mine	1964	242	24.0
Gunnlaugsson	1970	334	11.7
Bünte	1973	200	30.5
Eichfuss	1984	134	9.7
Suehiro	1984	103	3.8
Schulz	1984	217	8.8
Gall	1985	249	11.6
Günther	1985	188	6.3
Kujath	1986	63	4.7
Saario	1986	100	8.0
Siewert	1986	104	4.1
Walther	1986	151	9.3
Bittner	1987	137	2.2
Eigler	1987	97	6.2
Authors' Patients	1986	714	8.7

[a] Survey

great importance because of the observed high incidence of local recurrences following partial or subtotal distal gastrectomies. More recent reports have shown the percentage of R1 resections with tumor infiltration of the proximal resection margin to be as high as 20.[29,32-34]

More extended radical surgery is supposed to reduce the rate of recurrence and generally may improve survival rates at the same time. While logical from both a theoretical and clinical viewpoint, radical surgery was regarded as excessive therapy not dictated by oncologic requirements and which entailed additional perioperative risks with respect to complications, mortality, and morbidity. Furthermore, there was no evidence to demonstrate a clear improvement in prognosis.

A reconciliation of various therapeutic opinions over the past several years, however, was supported not only by retrospective counterarguments, but also by facts based on acquired knowledge and results. This is particularly true for postoperative risk, since the technique of total gastrectomy, including lymph-node dissection, has clearly improved because of increased experience.** In addition, more precise data and/or histopathologic criteria now exist with respect to various factors, ie, growth characteristics of the primary tumor as well as of metastatic patterns.[1,6,25,31-37]

Therefore it seems to be difficult to cite higher rates of complications or mortality and poor long-term results following total gastrectomy as primary arguments against its routine use (Table 1).*** For example, the incidence and

**Refs. 3, 5, 6, 13, 14, 19, 20, 22–24, 28, 29, 35.

***Refs. 1, 2, 3, 5, 10, 14, 19, 23, 24, 29.

mortality associated with insufficiency of the proximal anastomosis, one of the most frequent complications following total gastrectomy, can be reduced regardless of the performance of a hand-sutured or stapled anastomosis. The same holds true for morbidity, especially for pronounced reflux esophagitis with serious clinical impact. This complication may be largely prevented by appropriate selection of reconstruction procedures.

Without losing sight of the goal of improved prognosis, calculable or achieved survival rates can also be used to assess various therapeutic procedures. Resection approaches of more extended radicality with statistically poorer global results are comparatively different from stage-dependent gastrectomies with overall better survival rates following routine total gastrectomy.[3,14,16,18–20,22–24,29] The results of McNeer and associates[18] and Papachristou and Fortner[22] regarding tumor localization exclusively in the distal third of the stomach can be cited as examples. In addition to improved long-term results, their findings showed a decrease in the local recurrent ratio following, respectively, elective or extensive total gastrectomy.

The discrepancy between all comparisons of the results and the simultaneous difficulty involved in their interpretation and evaluation with respect to the argumentation for selecting the therapeutic procedure can only be explained by the fact that most reports are based on unicentric, historical analysis with variable patient selection, an imprecisely defined level of radicality, particularly as related to lymph-node dissection, and on stage or classifications which differ from one another most of the time.[3,17,33,37] The examinations of Schlag and Herfarth[38] and Gouzi and Paquet[39] (Table 2) may well be the sole exceptions. In cases utilizing a clearly defined study design or prospective planning, neither investigative group observed any significant increase in local recurrence or survival rates during various surgical procedures.

As mentioned previously, differing viewpoints or definitions regarding the extent of surgical procedure relate not only to the tumor-bearing organ, ie, the stomach, but also to lymphadenectomy and the issue of splenectomy. However, if lymph-node dissection is required as a basic condition for exact staging and a systematic radical approach,[1,12,28,35,37] not in the least because of the high inci-

Table 2. Results of a prospective study: total gastrectomy vs. subtotal distal gastrectomy in cases of antral carcinoma[a]

	Gastrectomy	Subtotal distal resection
Total (n)	76	93
Postoperative complications	34%	33%
Due to leaks of the anastomosis	3[b]	5[b]
Postoperative mortality	1 (1.3%)	3 (3.2%)
5-Year survival rate	49%	32%

[a] Gouzi JL, Paquet JC: Paper presented at the 32nd World Congress of Surgery, Sydney 1987, Abstract 344.
[b] Conservative treatment.

Table 3. Retrospective data on a comparison of results following total gastrectomy with and without extended (systematic) lymph-node dissection (review of literature)

		5-Year survival rate	
		Lymphadenectomy	
Author	Year	Limited (%)	Extended (%)
Mine	1970	10.1	21.4
Soga	1979	30.0	50.6
Kodama	1981	18.0	45.0[a]
Kodama	1981	18.0	39.0[b]
Ostertag	1984	75.0	92.0[c]

[a] With serous infiltration.
[b] With lymph-node metastases.
[c] Early gastric cancer only.

dence of false-negative and false-positive intraoperative classifications,[35] the results of a European and German survey must come as a surprise, regardless of the possibility of elevated risk of operation, potential changes in local immune response, or an increased occurrence of implantation metastases: systematic lymph-node extirpation is generally performed only in 27% and 44% of the cases in compartments I and II, respectively.[10,26] Although such a procedure seems likely to result in an improved prognosis, these results are based entirely on retrospective analyses (Table 3 and refs. 1,6,12,28,35). Obligatory splenectomy is performed only in 8 to 23% of all operations, owing to the potential for elevated risk of infection and altered immunology.[10,26] The frequency of splenectomy increases to approximately 70% when the cancer is located in upper parts of the stomach. With respect to the increased radicality of lymphadenectomy—especially in the hilus of the spleen—it seems realizable only when the left pancreas is simultaneously resected[28]; retrospective data overwhelmingly point to a possible improvement in prognosis without splenectomy.[9,13,28,30]

Our Experience

We have consistently performed routine gastrectomies, including systematic lymphadenectomy in compartments I and II, resection of the greater and lesser

Table 4. Malignant gastric tumors: authors' patients, 1968–1987

Total (n)	1825	
Early gastric carcinoma	152	(8.3%)
Advanced gastric carcinoma	1,358	(74.5%)
Recurrent carcinoma	147	(8.1%)
Carcinoma of the gastric remnant	85	(4.6%)
Nonepithelial, malignant tumors	83	(4.5%)

Table 5. Surgical procedures and clinical mortality for 1,510 early and advanced gastric carcinoma: authors' patients, 1968–1987

	Total		Postoperative mortality	
	n	%	n	%
Resection	1,135	75.2	120	10.6
Subtotal distal gastrectomy	313	20.7	40	12.8
Proximal gastrectomy	108	7.2	18	16.7
Total gastrectomy	714	47.3	62	8.7
Without resection	375	24.8	67	17.9
Exploratory laparotomy	230	15.2	35	15.2
Gastroenterostomy	58	3.8	13	22.4
Endoprosthesis	87	5.8	19	21.8
Total	1,510	100	187	12.4

omenta, and obligatory splenectomy since 1974, when data from clinical studies were lacking or nonexistent and definitions for histologically oriented approaches were imprecise and based solely on the aforementioned arguments. At this time subtotal distal gastrectomy was used primarily as a palliative procedure in patients with tumors localized in the antrum or with increased perioperative risks. This was the diagnosis in about 90% of the distal resections over the last 5 years, for example. Of a total 1825 malignant tumors the resection rate of 1510 early and advanced gastric carcinomas was 75% (Table 4); 714 total gastrectomies were carried out in addition to 313 subtotal distal and 108 proximal gastrectomies (Table 5).

The overall frequency of total gastrectomies under the resection procedure was 62.9% and rose in various time intervals from 25.2% to 67.9% and then to 81.1% over the last 5 years (Table 6). Clinical mortality of all resection procedures was 10.6%. A direct comparison of the mortality rates following subtotal distal (12.8%) and total gastrectomy (8.7%) reveals no statistically significant differences, even when various other parameters were specified and taken into account (Table 7). The high mortality rate following subtotal distal gastrectomy may be

Table 6. Distribution of resective procedures for 1,510 early and advanced gastric carcinoma over various time intervals: resection rate 75.2%, authors' patients, 1968–1987

	Type of resection					
	Subtotal distal gastrectomy		Proximal gastrectomy		Total gastrectomy	
Time interval	n	%	n	%	n	%
1968–1973	136	55.3	48	19.5	62	25.2
1974–1981	120	23.1	47	9.0	353	67.9
1982–1986	57	15.4	13	3.5	299	81.1
1968–1986	313	27.6	108	9.5	714	62.9

Table 7. Comparison of clinical mortality following subtotal distal gastrectomy and total gastrectomy for gastric carcinoma: authors' patients, 1968–1987

	Type of resection			
	Subtotal distal gastrectomy		Total gastrectomy	
Postoperative mortality	n	%	n	%
Total	40/133	12.8	62/714	8.7
1968–1973	22/136	16.2	11/62	17.7
1974–1981	11/120	9.2	30/353	8.5
1982–1986	7/57	12.3	21/299	7.0
Age ≤ 69 years	26/198	13.1	42/573	7.3
Age ≥ 70 years	14/115	12.1	20/141	14.2
Localization in middle and lower thirds of stomach	23/179	12.8	11/215	5.1
Prepyloric	3/47	6.4	0/25	–
Early stomach carcinoma	7/58	12.1	2/87	2.3
"Curative" total gastrectomy			28/411	6.8
"Palliative" total gastrectomy			34/303	11.2

attributed for the most part to the aforementioned unfavorable patient selection. In contrast, the morbidity and mortality rates could be generally reduced in the various time intervals following total gastrectomy; in the same manner insufficiency of an esophagojejunostomy with a resultant lethal outcome could be reduced (Table 8). The preferred reconstruction procedures performed in these cases were the jejunum interposition according to Longmire and the Roux-en-Y reconstruction; the proximal anastomosis was almost exclusively hand-sutured.

Analysis of survival rates showed that 22.6% of all operated patients lived for an additional 5 years; this was increased to 29.8% for all resection procedures and to 78.1% for early gastric carcinoma. Overall, no statistically significant differences were found among the various subtotal or total gastrectomies; when

Table 8. Clinical mortality, frequency of leakages of the proximal anastomosis following 714 gastrectomies for gastric carcinoma over various time intervals: authors' patients, 1968–1987

		Proximal anastomosis				Postoperative mortality total	
	Total	Total		Mortality			
	(n)	n	%	n	%	n	%
1968–1986	714	68	9.5	22	32.4	62	8.7
1968–1973	62	3	4.8	2	75.0	11	17.7
1974–1981	353	45	12.7	15	33.3	30	8.5
1982–1986	299	22	7.4	5	22.7	21	7.0

Table 9A. Survival rates after 1,510 operations for early and advanced gastric carcinoma (life table method,[a] including clinical mortality): authors' patients, 1968–1987

	Total (n)	Survival (% ± SE)	
		5 Years	10 Years
Early and advanced gastric carcinoma	1,510	22.6 ± 1.2	18.2 ± 1.2
Advanced carcinoma	1,358	16.4 ± 1.1	12.6 ± 1.0
Early carcinoma	152	78.1 ± 3.7	68.8 ± 4.7
Resections	1,135	29.8 ± 1.5	23.9 ± 1.5
Subtotal distal gastrectomy	313	33.2 ± 2.8	25.7 ± 2.7
Proximal gastrectomy	108	21.7 ± 4.1	15.5 ± 3.7
Total gastrectomy	714	30.5 ± 2.0	26.3 ± 2.0
"Curative" total gastrectomy	411	47.6 ± 2.9	41.3 ± 3.2
"Palliative" total gastrectomy	303	6.9 ± 1.6	6.3 ± 1.6
"Curative" total gastrectomy (from 1974)	377	49.3 ± 3.2	43.1 ± 3.5

[a] Cutler SJ, Ederer F: Maximum utilization of the life table method in analyzing survival. J Chron Dis 1958;8:699.

tumor localization and histomorphologic classification were considered, the renewed direct comparison between distal and total gastrectomy could not show any difference. The varying criteria for recruiting or selecting patients for a retrospective evaluation must be taken into account here as well. Nevertheless, the 5-year survival rate of approximately 50% following total gastrectomy classified as curative, as well as the stabilizing and rising trend witnessed in recent years, may be viewed as positive developments (Tables 9A and 9B).

Table 9B. Comparison of survival rates after subtotal distal gastrectomy and total gastrectomy for gastric carcinoma, taking into account localization and histologic tumor type (life table method,[a] including clinical mortality): authors' patients, 1968–1987

	Total (n)	Survival (% ± SE)	
		5 Years	10 Years
Localization: middle and distal third			
Subtotal distal gastrectomy	179	39.8 ± 3.7	31.3 ± 3.6
Total gastrectomy	215	50.5 ± 3.7	45.9 ± 3.9
Histology "intestinal"			
Subtotal distal gastrectomy	156	30.4 ± 4.1	23.3 ± 4.0
Total gastrectomy	246	29.0 ± 3.7	25.8 ± 3.8
Localization and histology: middle and distal thirds: "intestinal"			
Subtotal distal gastrectomy	85	34.1 ± 4.9	26.1 ± 4.7
Total gastrectomy	62	43.3 ± 7.3	39.9 ± 7.5

[a] Cutler SJ, Ederer F: Maximum utilization of the life table method in analyzing survival. J Chron Dis 1958;8:699.

Table 10. Surgical treatment of gastric carcinoma: literature review of survey results

Kieninger et al. (1982)[a]		
Survey in the FRG	208 centers, 6,023 patients	
	Total gastrectomy "de principe"	≈15%
	Total gastrectomy "preferred"	≈32%
	(66 of 208 centers)	
Raab et al. (1987)[b]		
Survey in the FRG	1,141 centers	
Nonuniversity centers	Total gastrectomy "preferred"	≈26%
University centers	Total gastrectomy "preferred"	≈22%
Günther et al. (1987)[c]		
Survey in Europe	62 centers, 16,594 patients	
	Total gastrectomy "de principe"	≈1.6%
		(1 of 62 centers)
For diffuse carcinoma	Total gastrectomy "preferred"	≈44%

[a] Kieninger G, Koslowski L, Kurz L, et al: Derzeitige operative Strategie beim Magencarcinom in Deutschland. Ergebnisse einer Umfrage, in Häring R (ed): Therapie des Magencarcinoms, med ed. Basel, Weinheim, 1984, p 95.

[b] Raab M, Godehardt E: Umfrage zur chirurgischen Behandlung des Magencarcinoms. Med Klin 1987;82:186.

[c] Günther B, Teichmann RK, Demmel N, et al: Aktuelle Chirurgie des Magencarcinoms. Mün med Wschr 1987;129:285.

Conclusions

The current situation of surgical therapy of gastric cancer has been demonstrated. We personally favor a treatment based on the obtained, but not statistically significantly proven, results.[3,20,23,24] Even though the interpretation of oncologic different, but not necessarily opposing, viewpoints and opinions has tended toward increasing reconciliation, the results of surveys regarding the surgical approach must be evaluated critically with respect to an adequate or sufficient radicality if the frequency of total gastrectomy as the preferred surgical procedure is only 20 to 40% (Table 10, refs. 10 and 26). This is even more surprising for a frequency of 60% of total gastrectomy, with regard to an exact definition and consequent execution of the histologically oriented procedure with respect to tumor classification leading to the subsequent observation of the oral margins of safety to be observed.[6] Once the definitions for such an approach are established and observed, those cases may quite accurately be described and quantitated for which a total gastrectomy is the operation of choice based on individual histomorphologically differentiated surgical procedure may represent an excessive therapy or may be demanded.

A precise evaluation and classification of our patients as part of a multicentric study show that when histologically oriented criteria are interpreted liberally, ie, in the presence of an intestinal type of carcinoma of the middle and lower third

Table 11. Tumor localization and histologic classification according to Laurén for 96 gastrectomies: portion of alternatively possible distal subtotal gastrectomy using a histologically oriented procedure: authors' patients (April 15, 1986–April 31, 1987)

	Histologic classification					
	"Intestinal"		"Diffuse"		Unclassified, mixed types	
Tumor localization	n	%	n	%	n	%
Broadly	2	2.1	1	1.0	1	1.0
Proximal third of stomach	31	32.3	6	6.3	3	3.1
Proximal/middle third of stomach	3	3.1 2°	3	3.1	1	1.0
Middle third of stomach	8	8.3	12	12.5 2°	–	–
Middle/lower third of stomach	2	2.1 1°	2	2.1	3	3.1
Lower third of stomach	6	6.3	12	12.5	–	–
Total	52	54.2	36	37.5	8	8.3

Postoperative mortality n = 1 (1.04%).
Portion of distal resections using a histologically oriented procedure.
1° = 6/96 (6.3%).
2° = 30/96 (31.3%).

of the stomach as well as a diffuse carcinoma of the distal stomach, a subtotal distal gastrectomy may be allowed in approximately 30% of cases. The subtotal distal gastrectomy would be an alternative to the performed total gastrectomy and sufficient from the standpoint of oncologic requirements as well. When these criteria for resection are further narrowed – ie, only taking into account intestinal antrum carcinomas – the number of possible alternative resection procedures is reduced to approximately 5% (Table 11); these results have increasingly stabilized in our data recently.[3]

Another decline in alternative resection procedures appears possible on the observation of epidemiologic data with drops in intestinal, distal gastric carcinomas given a simultaneous increase in the incidence of carcinomas of the esophagogastric junction without a rise in early tumor stages emerging.[1,2,4,29,33] Even if the evaluation parameters of primarily differing therapeutic arrangements seem to have become more objectifiable and intelligible, the requirement for clinical, multicenter (eg, interdisciplinary) studies remains as pressing as ever; this applies equally to examinations aimed at ascertaining the therapeutic and prognostic value of an expanded lymph-node dissection, as, for example, in compartment III[12,21,28,30,40] as well as to purely palliative surgical measures, particularly from the standpoint of the possible application of neoadjuvant therapy. Only under these circumstances the still primarily argumentatively supported initial and evaluative criteria can be proven or disproven by correspondingly valid results and without the well-known speculations.

References

1. Gentsch HH: Maligne Tumoren des Magens, in Gall FP, Hermanek P, Tonak J (eds): Chirurgische Onkologie. Berlin-Heidelberg-New York, Springer, 1986, p 347.
2. Hölscher AH, Siewert JR: Surgical treatment of adenocarcinoma of the gastrooesophageal junction. Dig Surg 1985;2:1.
3. Meyer H-J, Jähne J, Pichlmayr R: Magencarcinom: Gastrektomie de principe. Langenbecks Arch Chir 1987;372:571.
4. Meyers WC, Diaminano RJ, Rotolo FS, et al: Adenocarcinoma of the stomach. Ann Surg 1987;205:1.
5. Siewert JR, Ketterl R: Chirurgische Standortbestimmung: Magencarcinom. Z Gastroenterol 1985;29:100.
6. Gall FP, Hermanek P: New aspects in the surgical treatment of gastric carcinoma—a comparative study of 1636 patients operated on between 1969 and 1982. Eur J Surg Oncol 1985;11:219.
7. Gennari L, Bozetti F, Bonfanti G, et al: Subtotal versus total gastrectomy for cancer of the lower two thirds of the stomach: a new approach to an old problem. Br J Surg 1986;73:534.
8. Gilbertsen VA: Results of treatment of stomach cancer. Cancer 1969;23:1305.
9. Grundmann R, Weber F, Raab M: Splenektomie bei Gastrektomie? Eine Analyse der postoperativen Morbidität und des Patientenüberlebens. Akt Chir 1987;22:91.
10. Günther B, Teichmann RK, Demmel N, et al: Aktuelle Chirurgie des Magencarcinomsk. Mün med Wschr 1987;129:285.
11. Kieninger G, Koslowski L, Kurz L, et al: Derzeitige operative Strategie beim Magencarcinom in Deutschland. Ergebnisse einer Umfrage, in Häring R (ed): Therapie des Magencarcinoms, med ed. Basel, Weinheim, 1984, p 95.
12. Kodoma Y, Sugimachi K, Soejima K, et al: Evaluation of extensive lymph node dissection for carcinoma of the stomach. World J Surg 1981;5:241.
13. Lersch C, Schreiner J, Demmel N, et al: Monitoring immunocompetent cells in the peripheral blood of stomach cancer patients after splenectomy and gastrectomy. J Cancer Res Clin Oncol 1985;110:225.
14. Longmire WP: Total gastrectomy for carcinoma of the stomach. Surg Gynecol Obstet 1947;84:21.
15. Longmire WP: Gastric carcinoma: is radical gastrectomy worth while? Ann Roy Coll Surg Engl 1980;62:25.
16. Lortat-Jacob JL, Giuli R, Estenne B, et al: Intérèt de la gastrectomie totale pour le traitement des cancers de l' estomac. Chirurgie 1975;101:59.
17. Lundh G, Burn JI, Kolig G: A co-operative international study of gastric cancer. Ann Roy Coll Surg Engl 1974;54:219.
18. McNeer G, Bowden L, Booher RJ, et al: Elective total gastrectomy for cancer of the stomach: end results. Ann Surg 1974;180:252.
19. Merkle P: Ausdehnung und Taktik bei der operativen Therapie des Magencarcinoms. Klinikarzt 1978;7:381.
20. Meyer H-J, Pichlmayr R, Geerlings H: Die Gastrektomie als Regeloperation beim Magencarcinom, in Bünte H, Langhans P, Meyer H-J, et al (eds): Aktuelle Therapie des Magencarcinoms. Berlin-Heidelberg-New York, Springer, 1985, p 60.
21. Mishima Y, Hirayama R: The role of lymph node surgery in gastric cancer. World J Surg 1987;11:406.

22. Papachristou DN, Fortner JG: Choice of the operative procedure for adenocarcinoma of the gastric antrum. J Surg Oncol 1982;21:241.
23. Pichlmayr R, Meyer H-J: Value of the gastrectomy "de principe," in Herfarth C, Schlag P (eds): Gastric Cancer. Berlin-Heidelberg-New York, Springer, 1979, p 196.
24. Pichlmayr R, Meyer H-J: Indication for total gastrectomy. Nutrition, in publication.
25. Priesching A: Die Therapie des Magencarcinoms. Munich, Urban & Schwarzenberg, 1980.
26. Raab M, Godehardt E: Umfrage zur chirurgischen Behandlung des Magencarcinoms. Med Klin 1987;82:186.
27. Rush BF, Ravitch MM: The evaluation of the total gastrectomy. Inter Abstr Surg 1962;114:411.
28. Siewert JR, Lange J, Böttcher K, et al: Lymphadenektomie beim Magencarcinom. Langenbecks Arch Chir 1986;268:137.
29. Siewert JR, Lange J, Böttcher K, et al: Magencarcinom, Bestandsaufnahme aus chirurgischer Sicht. Dtsch med Wschr 1987;112:622.
30. Yoshino K, Haruyama K: Bedeutung der Splenektomie für die Lymphknotenausräumung beim Magencarcinom. Akt Chir 1983;18:81.
31. Inberg MV, Laurén P, Viikari SJ: Die Prognose des Magencarcinoms vom intestinalen Typ und vom diffusen Typ nach Magenresektion, in Beger HG, Bergemann W, Oshima H (eds): Das Magencarcinom. Stuttgart, Georg Thieme, 1980, p 247.
32. Bonzetti F, Bonfanti G, Bufalino R, et al: Adequacy of margins of resection in gastrectomy for cancer. Ann Surg 1982;196:685.
33. Cunningham D, Hole D, Taggart DJ, et al: Evaluation of the prognostic factors in gastric cancer: the effect of chemotherapy on survival. Br J Surg 1987;74:715.
34. Papachristou DN, Koras M, Fortner JG: Anastomotic recurrence in the oesophagus complicating gastrectomy for adenocarcinoma of the stomach. Br J Surg 1979;66:609.
35. Gall FP, Hermanek P: Indikation für die systematische Lymphknotendissektion beim Magenkarzinom, in Rohde H, Troidl H (eds): Das Magencarcinom. Stuttgart, Georg Thieme, 1984, p 158.
36. Cuschieri A: Gastrectomy for gastric cancer: definitions and objectives. Br J Surg 1986;73:513.
37. Hermanek P: Magencarcinom: chirurgische Pathologie, TNM-Systeme. Langenbecks Arch Chir 1982;358:57.
38. Schlag P, Herfarth C: Beziehung zwischen Ausdehnung des operativen Primäreingriffs und locoregionären Rezidiven, in Rohde H, Troidl H (eds): Das Magencarcinom. Stuttgart, Georg Thieme, 1984, p 138.
39. Gouzi JL, Paquet JC: Paper presented at the 32nd World Congress of Surgery, Sydney 1987, Abstract 344.
40. Keighley MRB, Moore J, Roginski C, et al: Incidence and prognosis of N4 node involvement in gastric cancer. Br J Surg 1984;71:863.

CHAPTER 6

Surgical Treatment of Gastric Cancer: Carcinomas of the Gastroesophageal Junction

A.H. Hölscher, M. Schüler, and J.R. Siewert

Introduction

Surgical therapy of gastroesophageal junction carcinomas is of special interest in the setting of the discussion on gastric carcinoma for two reasons. First, a relative increase in the so-called carcinoma of the cardia has been reported by authors from several countries in recent years.[1-5] This shift in the topography of gastric carcinoma, which has been described by Ottenjann in the German lingual sphere,[4] is also reproducible in the authors' patient group of the last 5 years. On the other hand, the selection of procedures for cardiac carcinoma is as controversial as its definition (Fig. 1). In a questionnaire submitted to 22 European surgical clinics with a total of 1,200 patients with cardiac carcinoma, seven variants concerning extent of resection alone were described.[6]

Some authors advocate total esophagogastrectomy,[7,8] others emphasize the necessity for principal gastrectomy,[9,10] and yet others[11] accept a restricted regional cardiac resection as satisfactory. Reasons for this therapeutic uncertainty include a lack of data on outcomes which can be achieved by the different procedures and the ambiguity of the term "cardiac carcinoma" in the literature.[11,12] However, as long as this term is used for many different types of tumors, results of treatment will be difficult to compare and clear therapeutic guidelines cannot be expected.

At the Surgical Clinic of the Technical University of Munich cardiac carcinoma is used to designate adenocarcinomas of the gastroesophageal junction – the area 5 cm orad and 5 cm caudad to the lower esophageal sphincter. Lower esophageal carcinomas and subcardiac gastric carcinomas are included in this category only if they infiltrate the cardia, ie, the terminal esophageal musculature. To narrow this definition further, the necessity for a thoracoabdominal or an abdomino-transhiatal procedure for radical tumor resection is regarded as second criterion.

If this definition is observed, the term cardiac carcinoma comprises three different types of adenocarcinomas (Fig. 2).

1. Adenocarcinoma in the endobrachyesophagus (Barrett's esophagus), as long as it develops within the borders mentioned (type I; Fig. 3A);

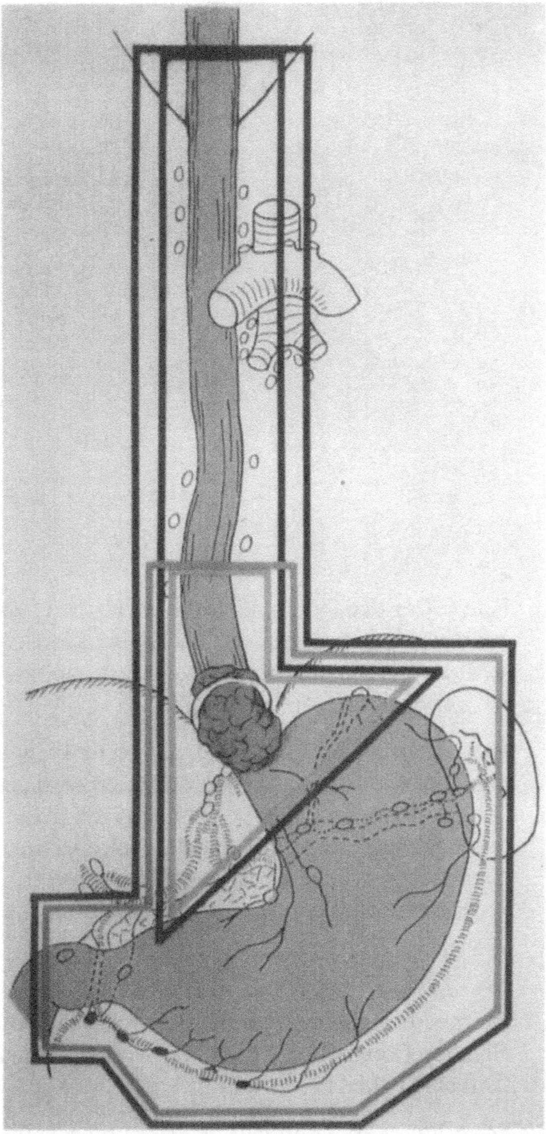

Fig. 1. Schematic of the various extents of resection in adenocarcinoma of the gastroesophageal junction: limited cardiac resection, lower esophageal resection and total gastrectomy, subtotal esophageal resection and proximal gastric resection, total esophagogastrectomy.

2. True cardiac carcinoma, emerging from the cardiac mucosa (type II; Fig. 3B);
3. Subcardiac or fundus carcinoma of the stomach, which infiltrates the lower esophagus mostly submucosally (type III; Fig. 3C).

These types of tumors require different surgical therapy. Our clinic in 1982 determined selection of procedure and extent of resection based in part on an analysis of the literature but largely by the retrospective analysis of 49 operated cardiac carcinomas, as follows.[13]

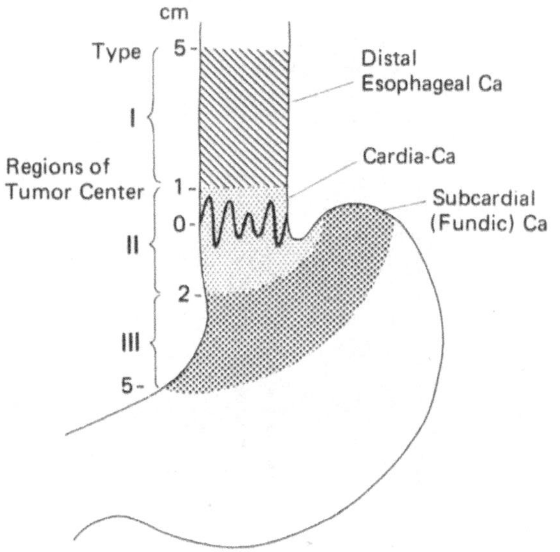

Fig. 2. Classification of the adenocarcinomas of the gastroesophageal junction. (Adapted, with permission, from Siewert JR, Hölscher AH, Becker K, et al: Cardiacarcinom: Versuch einer therapeutisch relevanten Klassifikation. Chirurg 1987;58:25.)

Type I: Cervicoabdominal transmediastinal subtotal esophagectomy, proximal gastrectomy (fundectomy), and lymphadenectomy of the so-called compartment II;[14] reconstruction of the intestinal passage per gastric tube formation and cervical anastomosis (Fig. 4).

Type II: In stage I/II[15] total gastrectomy with distal esophageal resection (thoracoabdominal) and reconstruction with pediculated esophagojejunoplication (Roux-en-Y)[16] or esophagojejunostomy with a stapled anastomosis.

In advanced stages III and IV, total gastrectomy and subtotal esophagectomy; reconstruction with colonic interposition (colon transversum perfused by the left colonic artery) with cervical anastomosis and coloduodenostomy (Fig. 4).

Type III: Thoracoabdominal or abdominotranshiatal total gastrectomy with lower esophageal resection, reconstruction with pediculated esophagojejunoplication (Roux-en-Y; Fig. 4) or esophagojejunostomy with stapled anastomosis (end-to-side).

Since July 1, 1982 all cardiac carcinomas which matched these criteria were prospectively recorded, documented, and worked up as a protocol with respect to pathoanatomy. The current examination of these protocols was directed to the question of whether this classification and the therapeutic consequences resulting thereof have proven valid in the light of critical analysis.

Methods

All patients were diagnosed preoperatively according to a fixed protocol. A large thoracic survey radiograph in two planes with contrast visualization of esophagus

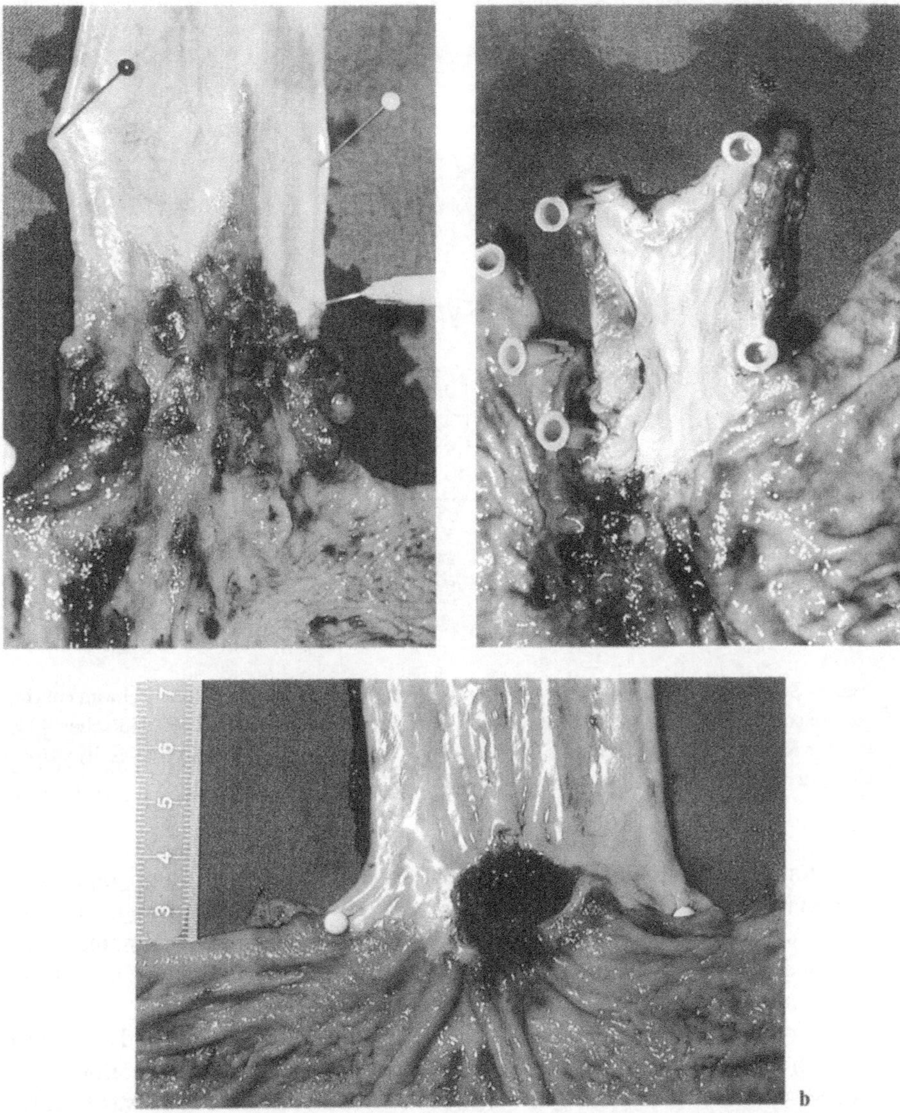

a c b

Fig. 3. (**A**) type I: adenocarcinoma in the Barrett's esophagus; (**B**) type II: adenocarcinoma of the cardiac mucosa; (**C**) type III: subcardiac adenocarcinoma.

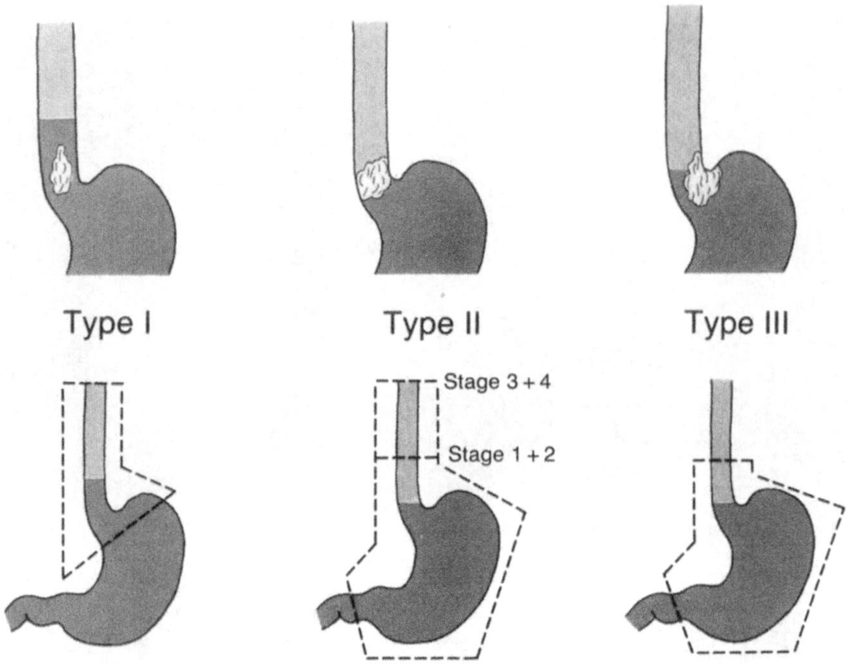

Fig. 4. Schematic display of the extent of resection in patients with adenocarcinoma of the gastroesophageal junction. (Adapted, with permission, from Siewert JR, Hölscher AH, Becker K, et al: Cardiacarcinom: Versuch einer therapeutisch relevanten Klassifikation. Chirurg 1987;58:25.)

and stomach (Thoramat x ray) was taken to localize the tumor topographically and anatomically (Fig. 5A–C). Thoramat x-rays were followed by a thoracic and upper abdominal CT scan and endoscopy. According to the findings thus obtained the individual carcinoma was designated preoperatively as one of the three tumor types.

This preoperative matching was also controlled intraoperatively and subject to correction. A surgical procedure was then selected according to the aforementioned scheme. After surgery an exact documentation of the tumor was filed by the surgeon on a corresponding formsheet, and every specimen was photographed. Subsequently xeromacrography and, following formalin fixation, another photographic documentation were performed at the Institute of Pathology.[17] After the tumor was measured, the pathologist classified it according to the aforedescribed scheme using macroscopic criteria, in particular tumor localization. Specimens were then worked up according to a prefixed protocol. Aside from the usual tumor diagnostics, examination of the specimen was carried out in 1-cm steps orad and aborad to determine tumor extension. Moreover, the lymph nodes, which were removed in the course of the lymphadenectomy, were prepared, counted, and examined histologically. In a final surgery-pathology

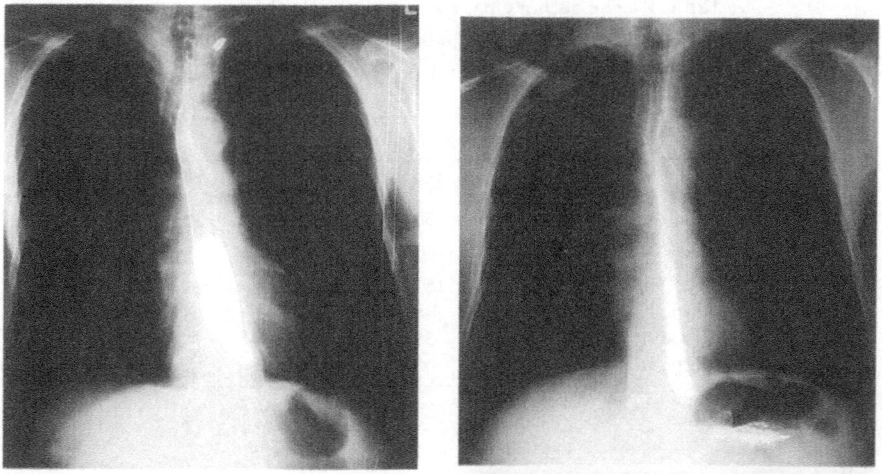

a b

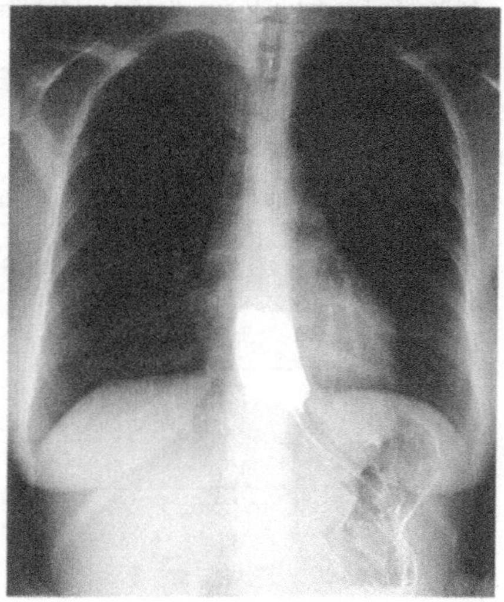

c

Fig. 5. Thoramat radiographs of patients with adenocarcinomas of the gastroesophageal junction. Topographical association of the tumor is greatly facilitated by the reference-points of the thorax. (**A**) type I; (**B**) type II; (**C**) type III. (Adapted, with permission, from Siewert JR, Hölscher AH, Becker K, et al: Cardiacarcinom: Versuch einer therapeutisch relevanten Klassifikation. Chirurg 1987;58:25.)

joint conference the association of all specimens was scrutinized once more by means of the tumor documentation, and possible discrepancies between clinical-surgical and pathoanatomic associations were resolved.

Patient Population

From July 1, 1982 to October 1, 1987 a total of 189 patients with adenocarcinoma of the gastroesophageal junction were admitted to the Surgical Clinic of the Technical University of Munich for treatment. Of these, 38 proved to be inoperable owing to their poor general medical condition (old age, distant metastases, etc) and were assigned to receive laser therapy and intraluminal afterloading radiation

Table 1. The authors' patient population with distribution of tumor types I–III in 151 patients with resected adenocarcinoma of the gastroesophageal junction (July 1, 1982–October 1, 1987)

	Number of patients	
Total	189	
Palliative treatment (Laser/Afterloading)	38	(Operation rate 80%)
Resection	151	(Resection rate 99.3%)
Type I	48	(32%)
Type II	38	(25%)
Type III	65	(43%)

Table 2. Epidemiologic characteristics and prevalence of Barrett's esophagus

	Age $\bar{x}$ (range)	Sex (M:F)	Barrett's esophagus
Type I	60 (29–74)	5:1	75%
Type II	55 (25–77)	4.5:1	5%
Type III	64 (31–78)	2.6:1	0%

Table 3. Tumor grouping stages I + II and III + IV in the authors' patient population[a]

Type	n	I + II pT_1-pT_2 $N_{0\text{-}1}$ M_0 (+ pT_3 N_0 M_0)	III + IV pT_3-pT_4 > N_1 M_X (+ pT_2 > N_2 M_0)
I	48	33.3%	66.7%
II	38	39.4%	60.6%
III	65	38.5%	61.5%
I–III	–	37.0%	63.0%

[a] From Hermanek P, Sobin LH: TNM-Classification of Malignant Tumors. UICC 4th ed. Berlin-Heidelberg-New York, Springer-Verlag, 1987, with permission.

Table 4. Average number of dissected lymph nodes with partition of involved lymph nodes correlated with type of tumor

Type	$\bar{x}$ Total	$\bar{x}$ Involved
I	36	14
II	38	11
III	43	14

Table 5. Frequency of lymph node metastases correlated with type of tumor (n ≥ 1): lymph nodes involved

Type I	77.1%
Type II	78.9%
Type III	76.9%

therapy. The remaining 151 patients – 80 % – with adenocarcinoma of the esophagogastric junction were operated on and resected as described initially. Except for one case, all patients who underwent surgery were resected as well; ie, the resection rate amounted nearly to 100%.

Results

The distribution of tumor types, based on the aforementioned criteria, is depicted in Table 1, according to the matching determined in the final clinical-surgical/pathoanatomic conference.

Epidemiologic characteristics and tumor stagings of these patients are presented in Tables 2 and 3, respectively. TNM assessment was based on the UICC classification, according to which the carcinomas operated on prior to 1987 were reclassified as well. To document lymph node metastasis into the various compartments individually, this classification was modified for N-stages in the following way:

For metastasis into the regional lymph nodes (compartment I according to the Japanese classification[18]), N1; for metastasis into compartment II, N2; and for metastasis into compartment III, N3. For adenocarcinoma of the lower esophagus (type I), thoracic and perigastric lymph nodes were evaluated as regional lymph nodes; for types II and III, as for example in gastric carcinoma, only the perigastric lymph nodes in compartment I (less than 3 cm). Frequency and distribution of lymph-node metastases are listed in Tables 4–6, and tumor infiltration into the orad and aborad margins of resection is shown in Table 7. Histologi-

Table 6. Involvement of various lymph node stations according to the TNM system correlated with tumor stage and type of carcinoma (analysis of 44 cases from October 1, 1986–October 1, 1987)

		pT_1–pT_2				pT_3–pT_4			
Type of carcinoma	n	N_0	N_1 (%)	N_2	N_3	N_0	N_1 (%)	N_2	N_3
I	12	25.0	16.7	0	–	8.3	50.0	0	–
II	15	33.3	13.3	20.0	–	–	6.7	26.7	–
III	17	29.4	23.5	11.8	–	–	5.9	17.0	11.8

Table 7. Tumor infiltration of the margin of resection in 151 adenocarcinomas of the gastroesophageal junction (including lymphangiosis carcinomatosa)

Type	n	Tumor at the orad margin of resection		Tumor at the aborad margin of resection	
I	48	2[a]	4.1%	1	2.1%
II	38	3[b]	7.8%	1	2.6%
		(Total Esophagogastrectomy: 0%)			
III	65	12[b]	18.4%	3	4.6%

[a] Cervical margin of resection.
[b] Margin of resection in distal esophageal resection.

cal results, which are important from a surgical point of view, are assembled in Fig. 6.

The results of surgical therapy were correlated with type of tumor (Table 8) and also analyzed according to surgical procedure (Table 9). Eventually the prognosis of the various types of tumors was determined by means of survival graphs (Fig. 7).

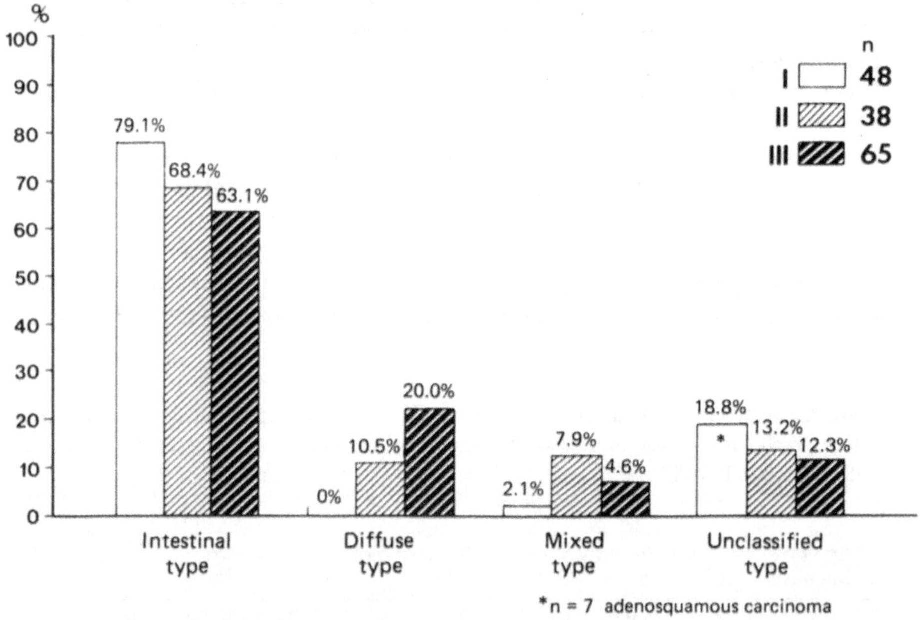

Fig. 6. Laurén classification and further histological differentiation of 151 patients with adenocarcinoma of the gastroesophageal junction.

Table 8. Results of surgical treatment in 151 patients with adenocarcinoma of the gastroesophageal junction correlated with type of tumor

Type	n	30-Day mortality		Hospital mortality	
I	48	4	8.3%	6	12.0%
II	38	2	5.2%	5	13.1%
III	65	2	3.1%	4	6.1%
I–III	151	8	5.2%	15	9.9%

Discussion

Reliability of Diagnostics and Classification

The uncertainty of definition and choice of procedure for cardiac carcinoma has prompted us to plan a prospective, observational study, guided by retrospective analysis of our patient population. Therefore, all adenocarcinomas of the gastroesophageal junction were prospectively registered, documented, and treated according to a fixed-therapy protocol, as long as the tumor centers could be located within 5 cm orad or aborad of the cardia. Matching to one of the three types of tumors was based on preoperative and operative diagnoses.

The Thoramat radiograph with concomitant barium visualization of esophagus and stomach has proven especially valuable for classification of the tumors. By means of these radiographs it has been possible in all cases to match the tumor, based on topographical and anatomical criteria, to one of the three types of tumors.

Although endoscopy provided important diagnostic information, this procedure provided less topographical/anatomical data than did radiography. Endo-

Table 9. Mortality in various types of surgical procedures in 151 patients with adenocarcinomas of the gastroesophageal junction. Slight changes of the figures in comparison to data in Table 8 are caused by the expansion of the procedure beyond the planned extent of resection for technical reasons and by discrepancies between preoperative-surgical and intra-postoperative pathoanatomic classification.

Surgical procedure	n	30-Day mortality		Hospital mortality	
Transmediastinal esophageal dissection	50	3	6.0%	5	10.0%
Total esophagogastrectomy	21	3	14.2%	3	14.2%
Lower esophageal resection + total gastrectomy	80	2	2.5%	7	8.7%
-Thoracoabdominal	50	1	2.0%	5	10.0%
-Abdominotranshiatal	30	1	3.5%	2	6.6%

scopy revealed vital evidence of endobrachyesophagus (Barrett's esophagus) and mucosal metastases in the esophagus. Moreover, the submucosal extension of a tumor could be assessed by retrograde inspection of the cardia. Classification of the adenocarcinoma via endoscopy was also undertaken.

CT and nuclear magnetic resonance contributed little to the classification of cardiac tumors. Their informational merit mainly concerned the extraluminal tumor extension and the detection of lymph node and distant metastases. Diagnostic validity amounted to only approximately 70%.[19]

Based on these preoperative diagnoses, in all cases a preoperative classification of the cardiac carcinoma was made by the surgeon most experienced in their treatment. This diagnosis was scrutinized intraoperatively by means of the situs. Intraoperative correction of the classification was necessary only in four (2.5%) cases, demonstrating a high reliability of preoperative classification according to radiological and endoscopic evidence.

Eventually the tumors were reclassified and worked up according to pathoanatomic criteria following a given protocol without direct knowledge of the matching by the surgeon. Therefore, macroscopic localization of the tumor center was taken for the decisive factor for classification. In discussing the pathoanatomic classification with the surgeons, correction of the clinical matching was necessary in 3.3% of cases.

A more detailed analysis of the patient data revealed no difference in age distribution and tumor stages. It is noteworthy that adenocarcinomas of the lower esophagus (type I) and true cardiac carcinoma (type II) occurred more frequently in the male patients of our population, a finding that has been confirmed by others.[3,20]

The therapeutic schedule for the various types of adenocarcinomas is shown in Fig. 4. Therapeutic outcomes not corresponding to this scheme were taken in only 4% of cases because of incorrect pre- or intraoperative classifications. The objective of the present analysis was to scrutinize the accuracy of the classification and its therapeutic consequences. Of primary importance was whether the extent of resection chosen could ensure absence of tumor from the intraluminal margins of resection.

Pathoanatomic Results

Histological examination of the resection specimens proved radicality concerning intraluminal tumor extension in 94% for type I, 90% for type II, and 80% for type III.

Adenocarcinoma in the Endobrachyesophagus (Barrett's Esophagus): Type I

Lymphangiosis carcinomatosa occurred on the cervical margin of resection in two patients with advanced type I tumors, proving the necessity for subtotal esophagectomy for type I carcinoma. In a high percentage of cases, type I carcinoma tends to spread tumor within the submucosa or in the lymph tract of the esophageal wall. In one case the caudad margin of resection was infiltrated due to a T4 tumor, which was resected only palliatively. In all other cases, no tumor could be identified so that the caudad border of resection within the upper third of the stomach could be regarded as adequate. Lymphadenectomy in this procedure almost entirely comprises compartment II (with the exception of part of the lymph nodes in the hepatoduodenal ligament-sparing of the origin of the right gastric artery). In contrast, compartment I is taken into consideration only in the upper third of the stomach (preservation of the right gastric and the right gastroepiploic arteries). Thus, lymphadenectomy is less radical than for total gastrectomy (see below) but takes into consideration the main lymph draining tract of the type I carcinoma along the left gastric artery toward the celiac axis. Intraoperative revision of the lymph nodes retained and their biopsy did not detect tumor in any case.

Examination of involved lymph node stations of a group of 44 patients showed no N2 metastasis in type I carcinoma, implying that in this limited number of cases, the dissected compartment II was never affected by metastases. However, particularly advanced tumor stages in a high percentage of cases metastasized to the lymph node station N1, ie, the regional groups of lymph nodes, especially periesophageally. These facts prove once more that adenocarcinoma in the endobrachyesophagus must be considered an esophageal carcinoma and treated accordingly.

Subcardiac Carcinoma: Type III

The intraoperative evaluation concerning the orad margin of resection had to be corrected in 20% of cases, in which insufficient radicality is related primarily to a high portion of intentional palliative resections. However, it must be taken into account that the procedures with a transhiatal approach were performed with a favorable mortality of merely 3.5% in 30 patients (Table 4).

The pathoanatomic analysis of tumor spreading aborad showed that, with the exception of three cases of advanced diffuse carcinoma, a more or less extensive portion of the stomach was free of tumor in all other cases and theoretically could have been spared. In our opinion, however, preservation of the lower stomach with respect to the antrum does not result in any functional advantages for the patient.

On the contrary, direct anastomosis of a lower gastric remnant located intraabdominally with the esophagus leads to poor functional long-term results (high rate of alkaline reflux esophagitis). Moreover, radicality of lymphadenectomy is greater in total gastrectomy than in proximal partial resection (need for preservation of the right gastroepiploic artery as well as the right gastric artery [see above]).

Exact analysis of the number of lymph nodes in our data revealed an average of 32 lymph nodes in total gastrectomy (compartments I and II) but only 20 lymph nodes in proximal gastrectomy (compartment II, partially compartment I). In our opinion, both arguments favor total gastrectomy, and therapy therefore corresponds to that for gastric carcinoma. Although Papachristou and Fortner[10] come to the same conclusion on the basis of survival rates, their argumentation is not quite convincing because their data are derived from a retrospective analysis in which extent of lymphadenectomy has not been described. That the differing survival times after proximal total gastrectomy were due to a different extent of lymph node dissection therefore cannot be excluded.

True Cardiac Carcinoma: Type II

The occasional recommendation for total esophagogastrectomy—the most radical intraluminal therapeutic concept—in the case of true cardiac carcinoma is largely justified. In all resection specimens of this extent the margins of resection were free of tumor. On the other hand, total esophagogastrectomy is associated with a higher surgical risk than both of the other techniques (see Table 4), and postoperative sequelae must be taken into account. Therefore, we employ this invasive procedure only when no other is feasible, as with advanced cardiac tumors type II (stages III and IV).[15] In this case reconstruction within the tumor bed should be avoided, because of possible local recurrence, and reconstruction in the anterior mediastinum with cervical anastomosis is preferred. Only in such cases—exactly one half of our patients—did we decide in favor of total esophagogastrectomy.

We have treated smaller type II cardiac carcinomas (stages I and II) in the same way as subcardiac carcinomas, ie, based on the considerations presented. They were brought either to total gastrectomy or to lower esophageal resection. Distribution of lymph node metastases in type II in early relatively advanced tumor stages shows involvement of the N2 lymph node group in 20% to 27%, indicating that radical dissection of the compartment II is of special importance in this type of carcinoma. Postoperatively, tumor infiltration into the orad margin of resection occurred in three cases due to a discontinuous lymphangiosis carcinomatosa despite intraoperative frozen section examinations. This observation has led us to investigate the extent of resection in early tumor stages in a randomized study. By means of this the transmediastinal subtotal esophageal resection and proximal gastric resection will be compared to the procedure currently performed—lower esophageal resection and total gastrectomy.

Extraluminal spread of tumor was determined by the tumor stage. In the principally executed standardized lymphadenectomy, lymph node metastases were found in 77.5% of cases (type I: 77.1%; type II: 78.9%; type III: 76.9%). In addition to the pathoanatomic findings, 37% of resections could be registered as curative (stages I and II) and, correspondingly, 63.4% of cases as palliative (stages III and IV) (Table 3).

According to the pathoanatomic work-up of the surgical specimen, our classification and the extent of resection based thereupon have proven sufficient (R0-resection) in 88% of cases. Lymphangiosis carcinomatosa could be demonstrated relatively frequently on the cephalad margin of resection in the extended transabdominal-transhiatal gastrectomies. Because of this, these procedures are being performed abdomino-right thoracically or by means of an EEA toward the mediastinum, as these provide a larger safety margin in the region of the esophagus. All in all, the proposed classification appears reasonable and therapeutically relevant to us.

Results of Surgical Therapy

The rate of resection in the patient population presented here is very high—approximately 100%—and is nearly matched only in series of Ellis and Maggs[21] (74%) and Brookes and associates[22] (79.8%). It is notably lower in most other published data (42%, Sasse and associates[11]; 46%, Allum and associates[23]; 50%, Orel and associates[24]). It must be emphasized that in our patient population inoperability could always be determined before surgery, ie, that with one exception, all patients who were operated on could be resected as well. Therapeutic results in terms of postoperative mortality are comparable to published data (Table 5).[6] Mortality is increased if subtotal esophagectomy becomes necessary, as in type I or advanced type II tumors. It appears important that the mortality of type II carcinomas in clinical stages I and II, which were resected to a limited extent, was nil, in contrast to mortality of the advanced stages—10%—in which

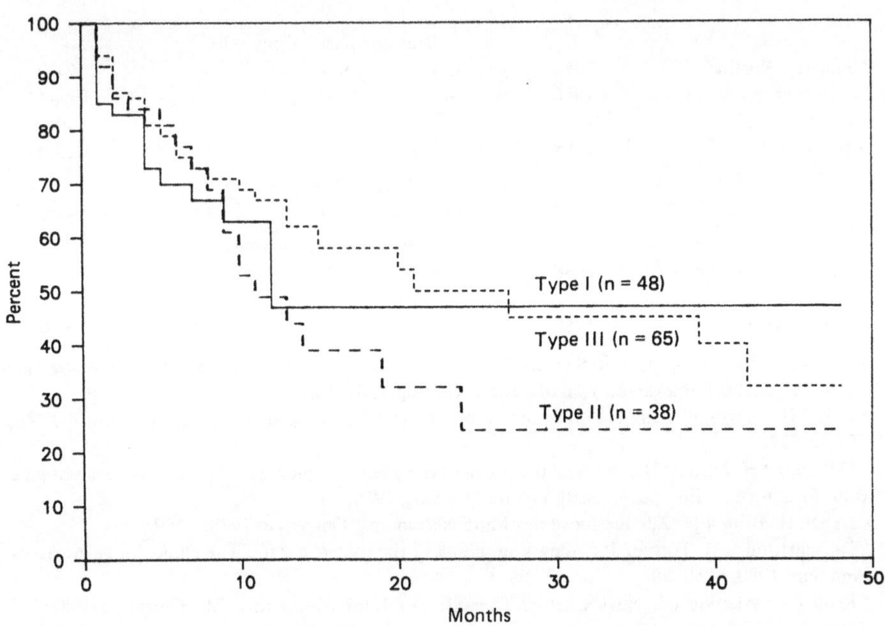

Fig. 7. Survival time correlated with tumor type (according to Kaplan EL, Meier P: Nonparametric estimates from incomplete observations. J Am Stat Assoc 1958;53:457). The differences among the three groups were not significant.

Table 10. Hospital mortality and survival rates of surgical treatment of adenocarcinomas of the gastroesophageal junction (cardiac carcinoma): compilation of the literature.

Investigators	Year	No. of patients	Hospital mortality (%)	2-Year survival rate (%)	5-Year survival rate (%)
Ellis, Maggs[a]	1946–1963	367	12.3	–	11.0
Ellis, Maggs[a]	1970–1980	42	2.4	–	11.1
Ellis, Maggs[a] (Lit. Comp)	1975–1980	1280	9.0	–	17.4
GEEMO[b] (Questionnaire)	1985	1200	11.9	33.6	14.8
Denck, Pridun[c]	1978	130	26.1	18.0	10.0
Papachristou, Fortner[d]	1980	101	15.0	–	12.0
Reding[e]	1982	45	15.5	–	13.3
Sasse, Bünte, Heinicke[f]	1985	80	16.2	45.0	26.0
Allum et al[g]	1986	265	19.0	26.8	9.8
			Radical resection		
		75	36.0	9.9	–
			Palliative resection		
Bolognese et al[h]	1988	137	25.5	–	22.0
Finley, Hobson, Duff[i]	1988	57	1.8	44.8	–
Orringer et al.[j]	1988	29	14.0	–	–
			Transthoracic resection		
		43	7.0	–	–
			Transmediastinal resection		
Hennessy, Keeling[k]	1988	128	19.4	–	24.0
Hernandez et al[l]	1988	47	17.0	–	–
Kakegawa et al[m]	1988	159	2.0	–	40.0
Valente et al[n]	1988	56	15.0	–	10.0
			Esophagogastrostomy		
		112	5.0	–	45.0
			Esophagojejunostomy		
Moreno-Gonzalez et al.[o]	1988	49	12.6	50.0 (3-year)	–
Authors' results	1988	151	9.9	44.0	33.0

Adapted, with permission, from Siewert JR, Hölscher AH, Becker K, et al: Cardiacarcinom: Versuch einer therapeutisch relevanten Klassifikation. Chirurg 1987;58:25.

[a] Ellis FH, Maggs PR: Surgery for carcinoma of the lower esophagus and cardia. World J Surg 1981;5:527.

[b] Hölscher AH, Siewert JR: Surgical treatment of the adenocarcinoma of the gastroesophageal junction. Results of an European questionnaire. Dig Surg 1985;2:1.

[c] Denck H, Pridun N: Zur Prognose des Kardiakarzinoms. Onkologie 1978;1:197.

[d] Papachristou DM, Fortner JS: Adenocarcinoma of the gastric cardia. The choice of gastrectomy. Ann Surg 1980;192/1:58.

[e] Reding R: Analyse der chirurgischen Therapie des Kardiakarzinoms. Zbl Chirurgie 1982;107: 1509.

[f] Sasse W, Bünte H, Heinicke A: Zur Prognose des Kardiacarcinoms. Langenbecks Arch Chir 1985; 365:205.

total esophagogastrectomy was required. However, net mortality was 14.2%, as an additional gastric resection with reconstruction by means of colon was necessary for technical reasons in one type I tumor.

Esophagogastrectomy is therefore a relatively high-risk procedure, and the indication to operate must be carefully considered in advanced cardiac carcinomas. Similar results (mortality of 12.6%) for total esophagogastrectomy have been reported by Moreno-Gonzalez and associates[25] for a comparable patient population. The analysis of survival in the various types of tumors also appears to confirm our conclusions (Fig. 7). Choice of procedure has not impaired the prognosis of any of these types of tumors as a consequence of insufficient resection. The slightly more favorable prognosis of the type I carcinoma is probably related to a relative accumulation of intestinal types of tumors (Fig. 6). Survival of patients with cardiac carcinomas in our series corresponded to published results (Table 10).

In conclusion, classification of adenocarcinoma of the esophagogastric junction with subdivision into adenocarcinoma of the endobrachyesophagus (Barrett's esophagus), true cardiac carcinoma, and subcardiac gastric carcinoma has proven useful. Preoperative matching can be achieved by radiography and endoscopy with a high degree of reliability. The classification permits the determination of an adequate extent of resection and thus can lower surgical risk. Total

---

[g] Allum WH, Roginski C, Fielding JWL, et al: Adenocarcinoma of the cardia: a 10-year review. World J Surg 1986;10:462.

[h] Bolognese A, Chirletti P, Sanmartino P, et al: Surgical treatment of carcinoma of the gastroesophageal junction. An analysis of 215 cases, in Siewert JR, Hölscher AH (eds): Diseases of the Esophagus. Berlin-Heidelberg-New York, Springer, 1988, p 582.

[i] Finley RJ, Hobson J, Duff J: Esophagogastrectomy without thoracotomy for adenocarcinoma of the cardia and lower esophagus, in Siewert JR, Hölscher AH (eds): Diseases of the Esophagus. Berlin-Heidelberg-New York, Springer, 1988, p 586.

[j] Orringer MB, Goldfaden D, Appelman HD, et al: Adenocarcinoma of the distal esophagus and gastric cardia. Comparison of results of transhiatal esophagectomy and thoracoabdominal esophagogastrectomy, in Siewert JR, Hölscher AH (eds): Diseases of the Esophagus. Berlin-Heidelberg-New York, Springer, 1988, p 599.

[k] Hennessy TPJ, Keeling P: Adenocarcinoma of the esophagus and cardia, in Siewert JR, Hölscher AH (eds): Diseases of the Esophagus. Berlin-Heidelberg-New York, Springer, 1988, p 579.

[l] Hernandez F, Suarez A, Torres AJ, et al: Surgical treatment in cancer of the cardia, in Siewert JR, Hölscher AH (eds): Diseases of the Esophagus. Berlin-Heidelberg-New York, Springer, 1988, p 611.

[m] Kakegawa T, Takeda J, Hashimoto K, et al: Thoraco-abdominal approach as a routine procedure for adenocarcinoma of the gastroesophageal junction, in Siewert JR, Hölscher AH (eds): Diseases of the Esophagus. Berlin-Heidelberg-New York, Springer, 1988, p 603.

[n] Valenté M, Pastorino U, Aloisio M, et al: Antrum versus gastric tube after partial esophagogastrectomy for adenocarcinoma of the gastric cardia, in Siewert JR, Hölscher AH (eds): Diseases of the Esophagus. Berlin-Heidelberg-New York, Springer, 1988, p 607.

[o] Moreno-Gonzalez E, Gomez Gutierrez M, Landa Garcia I, et al: Total extended esophagogastrectomy without thoracotomy as surgical treatment of the cardia, in Siewert JR, Hölscher AH (eds): Diseases of the Esophagus. Berlin-Heidelberg-New York, Springer, 1988, p 589.

esophagectomy in this therapeutic concept remains reserved for the advanced true cardiac carcinoma (type II). The extent of resection in early tumor stages of the type II will be examined in a prospective study.

References

1. Cady B, Choe DS: Changing patterns of gastric cancer. Trans 3rd Int Sym Detection and Prevention of Cancer. 1977:2041.
2. Antonioli DA, Goldman H: Changes in the location and type of gastric adenocarcinoma. Cancer 1982;50:775.
3. Kalish RJ, Clancy PE, Orringer MB, et al: Clinical, epidemiologic and morphologic comparison between adenocarcinomas arising in Barrett's esophageal mucosa and in the gastric cardia. Gastroenterology 1984;86:461.
4. Ottenjann R: Relative Zunahme des Cardiacarcinomas? Dtsch med Wschr 1984; 109:1303.
5. Paterson IM, Easton DF, Corbishley CM, et al: Changing distribution of adenocarcinoma of the stomach. Br J Surg 1987;74:481.
6. Hölscher AH, Siewert JR: Surgical treatment of the adenocarcinoma of the gastroesophageal junction. Results of an European questionnaire. Dig Surg 1985;2:1.
7. Giuli R, Gignoux M: Treatment of carcinoma of the esophagus. Ann Surg 1980;192:44.
8. Kunath V, Joka T: Überlegungen zur Operationstaktik beim Adenocarcinom der Cardia. Dtsch med Wschr 1983;108:94.
9. Kock NG: Chirurgische Behandlung von Oesophagus- und Kardiakrebs. Chirurg 1972;43:493.
10. Papachristou DM, Fortner JS: Adenocarcinoma of the gastric cardia. The choice of gastrectomy. Ann Surg 1980;192/1:58.
11. Sasse W, Bünte H, Heinicke A: Zur Prognose des Kardiacarcinoms. Langenbecks Arch Chir 1985;365:205.
12. Siedeck M: Die chirurgische Therapie des Kardiacarcinoms. Therapiewoche 1981;31:295.
13. Siewert JR, Weiser HF, Schattenmann G: Resektion von Cardia und distalem Oesophagus von rechts, in Häring R (ed): Chirurgie des Oesophaguscarcinoms, Edition Medizin. Deerfield Beach-Basel-Weinheim, 1981, p. 107.
14. Siewert JR, Lange J, Böttcher K, et al: Lymphadenektomie beim Magencarcinom. Langenbecks Arch Chir 1986;368:137.
15. Hermanek P, Sobin LH: TNM-Classification of Malignant Tumors. UICC, 4th ed. Berlin-Heidelberg-New York, Springer, 1987.
16. Siewert JR, Hölscher AH: Operationsverfahren beim Carcinom des gastrooesophagealen Ubergangs, in Bünte H, Langhans P, Meyer HJ, et al (eds): Aktuelle Therapie des Magencarcinoms. Berlin-Heidelberg-New York, Springer, 1985.
17. Schüler M: Rationelle Methode zur Makrodokumentation von Operatiospräparaten. Pathologie 1987;8:250.
18. Japanese Research Society for Gastric Cancer: The general rules for the gastric cancer study in surgery and pathology. Jpn J Surg 1981;11:127.
19. Lehr L, Rupp N, Reiser M, et al: Preoperative evaluation of resectability of esophageal cancer by CT- and MR-imaging, in Siewert JR, Hölscher AH (eds): Diseases of the Esophagus. Berlin-Heidelberg-New York, Springer, 1988, p. 146.

20. Sons HV, Borchard F: Cancer of the distal esophagus and cardia. Incidence, tumorous infiltration and metastatic spread. Ann Surg 1986;203/2:188.
21. Ellis FH, Maggs PR: Surgery for carcinoma of the lower esophagus and cardia. World J Surg 1981;5:527.
22. Brookes VS, Waterhouse JAH, Powell DJ: Carcinoma of the stomach: a 10-year survey of results and of factors affecting prognosis. Br Med J 1965;1:1577.
23. Allum WH, Roginski C, Fielding JWL, et al: Adenocarcinoma of the cardia: a 10-year review. World J Surg 1986;10:462.
24. Orel JJ, Erzen JJ, Hrabar BA: Results of resection for carcinoma of the esophagus and cardia in 196 patients. World J Surg 1981;5:295.
25. Moreno-Gonzalez E, Gomez Gutierrez M, Landa Garcia I, et al: Total extended esophagogastrectomy without thoracotomy as surgical treatment of the cardia, in Siewert JR, Hölscher AH (eds): Diseases of the Esophagus. Berlin-Heidelberg-New York, Springer, 1988, p. 589.

CHAPTER 7

The Surgical Treatment of Gastric Carcinoma: Possibilities for Palliative Treatment

G. Feifel and G. Schüder

Introduction

The surgical removal of gastric carcinoma continues to be the only method of treatment that offers the afflicted patient a chance for healing or improvement of symptoms. Unfortunately, however, the number of advanced tumors for which no chance of healing exists remains high, making palliative procedures of great importance in surgical practice.

Description and Problem Definition

The term "palliative tumor therapy" defines various treatment principles, as discussed below.

Palliation in a Narrower Sense

Curative surgery is either no longer possible or no longer makes sense given the advanced stage of the tumor (eg, T4 or Ml). The objective of a planned palliative measure is to eliminate or reduce symptoms such as dysphagia, vomiting, bleeding, and pain resulting from obstruction (eg, pyloric stenosis), oncolysis, and tumor infiltration. Emergency operations due to profuse bleeding or tumor perforation also fall into this category. Palliative surgical intervention may also help, at least indirectly, prolong life.[1]

Palliation from the Standpoint of Oncology

The planned surgical objective cannot be achieved. Surgery is commenced with the objective of cure, but ends up as palliative, since tumor tissue is left behind or has to be left behind macroscopically or microscopically.

Clinical Consequences

It is possible that the operability or resectability of the stomach cannot be determined with absolute certainty, despite the application of modern diagnostic procedures. The number of false-positive and false-negative prognoses of tumor expansion (eg, via computer tomography) is too high to set up a reliable plan of surgical treatment.[2] Endosonography seems to enable a reliable prognosis of resectability. Sufficiently broad experience has yet to be gathered, however.[3] The upshot is that the definitive decision regarding surgical procedure may be reached only during surgery, following careful exploration of the abdominal cavity. A considerable number of palliative operations are correctly recognized as such only after a work up of the specimen obtained. Checking the resection edges via an immediate section for microscopic examination during surgery therefore represents an important step. Intraoperative stage classification by the surgeon may be very difficult. Informative in this regard is the study by Madden,[4] which points to the poor agreement between intraoperative and histological examinations.

The R classification (UICC 1983) has been proven effective for the assessment of curability:

R0: No residual tumor. Resection lines and resection surfaces histologically free of tumor.
R1: Microscopically detectable residual tumor.
R2: Macroscopically discernible tumor, whether local or in the form of lymph-node metastases.

Most of the published literature puts the share of palliative resections at between 30% and 40%.[5-7] The curative/palliative/exploratory ratio in a group of 100 patients consecutively operated on in these cases was 44:40:16. Every third patient underwent a palliative resection (Table 1).

Table 1. Percentage of palliative resections in cases of gastric carcinoma

	Total		Resections		Palliative		GE/ Exploratory laparotomy	
Author	Year	n	n	%	n	%	n	%
Sasse	1985	853	493	57.1	105	21.3	360	42.2
Scott	1985	180	137	76.1	57	41.6	43	23.9
Siewert	1987	359	307	85.5	117	38.9	52	14.5
Cunningham	1987	277	160	57.7	32	20.0	117	42.3
Our results	1987	100	76	76.0	32	32.0	24	24.0

Siewert JR, Lange J, Böttcher K, et al: Magenkarzinom-Bestandsaufnahme aus chirurgischer Sicht. *Dtsch Med Wschr* 1987;112:622. Reprinted with permission of Georg Thieme Verlag, Stuttgart.

The most frequent intraoperative false diagnosis is encountered for large tumors projecting over the walls, which are mistakenly classified by the operating surgeon as T4.[8] The size of a tumor per se does not enable conclusions regarding curability. Immediate intraoperative sections for microscopic examination during surgery can be clarifying in these cases as well.[9]

Indications for Palliative Surgery and Range of Methods

A particularly painstaking assessment of benefits and risks is required for deciding whether to proceed with palliative surgery.[1,10-13] Only severe symptoms such as signs of stenosis and bleeding may be improved effectively by means of a palliative resection. No surgical procedure will lead to an improvement in the condition of asymptomatic, cachectic patients and in patients with tumor pains induced by infiltration. Additionally, the surgeon's experience is an important factor in the indication for surgery. The substantial drop in the death rate due to surgery which took place in recent years makes it possible to carry out a palliative tumor removal in older patients as well. In contrast, simultaneous surgical interventions into the abdominal and thoracic cavities are hardly ever justified. Emergency indications such as severe or recurring bleeding from a tumor at the esophagogastric junction occasionally mandate surgical reconstruction of the passage using bypass operations.[11,14]

In rare cases of tumor-induced gastric perforation an attempt should be made to remove the tumor in one operation.[15] Possibilities for palliative treatment encompass the entire gamut of standard gastric operations and, in cases of nonresectable proximal tumors, endoscopic procedures such as feeding tubes, bougienage, tube implantation, and laser coagulation. Even if a generally valid statement about these methods—which are still being tested—cannot yet be expressed, there is no doubt that the much smaller endoscopic surgical intervention places less of a burden on many patients than does a laparotomy.

Surgical Risk and Course

On an international level, the TNM tumor classification simultaneously symbolized the most important prognostic factors of gastric carcinoma. The consensus experience has been that the fate of a patient with a gastric tumor depends on the extent of tumor penetration (T), lymph-node status (N), and on the absence or detection of distant metastases (M).[16]

Patients who undergo a palliative procedure either have an advanced tumor or are in such poor condition overall that radical surgery is no longer an option. As the results of numerous reports show, the risk of surgery correlates with the local findings and general condition more than it does with the extent of the surgical treatment. This explains the high hospital mortality rate for relatively minor operations such as gastroenterostomy (Table 2).

Table 2. Clinical death rate for curative and palliative surgical procedures in cases of gastric carcinoma

	Total	Mortality	
Type of treatment	n	n	%
Gastrectomy	529	55	10.4
Resection			
Distal	386	28	7.1
Proximal	75	13	18.3
Exploratory laparotomy	194	20	9.6
Gastroenterostomy	83	21	23.3
Various	96	14	16.2
No surgery	60	7	11.1

Rohde H, Rau E, Gebbensleben B, et al: What causes in-hospital mortality of surgical patients with cancer of the stomach? *Scand J Gastroenterol* 1987;22(suppl 133):76. Reprinted with permission.

Since the death rate for palliative surgery with retained tumor is virtually the same as that for an exploratory laparotomy, gastroenterostomy is almost unanimously rejected.[5,8,10,13,17] Retrospective analysis tells us that the course and survival time are better after palliative tumor removal and should therefore be the primary focus of efforts. This was also confirmed in our patients (Table 3). Survival time may be increased significantly following palliative resection compared to the natural course of the disease.[10,13,18,19]

The decision regarding type of palliative procedure cannot be based only on statistical and empirical performance figures. The principle behind treatments according to the stage must be supplemented by a patient-oriented attitude. Usually of such utmost importance, the concept of survival time loses its significance in favor of a bearable period of life under certain circumstances when the surgery is no longer curative. This means that palliative procedures must be geared especially toward the individual situation as well as the opinion of the respective patient. This is naturally a demanding requirement which is occasionally difficult to implement in practice.

Table 3. Clinical mortality for 100 consecutive patients with gastric carcinoma in 1986–1987, average age 62.4 ± 11.3 years

	Total	Clinical mortality	
Operation	n	n	%
Tumor removal			
Curative	44	34	9.0
Palliative	32	65	15.6
Tumor remnant (eg, gastroenterostomy)	8	3	37.7
Exploratory laparotomy	16	5	31.3

The definition for the concept of quality of life must in this connection be expanded. The description of this concept is inadequate if restricted only to the restoration of function and elimination of disease. While this established and always debated definition does represent an important final end in the assessment of surgical procedures, it offers insufficient help to the incurable patient in terms of his most serious problem. Quality of life in a broader context would be a scenario in which the patient could come to terms with his disease as well as determine and accept the scope of remaining options contingent on the situation.[20]

A difficult conflict often emerges already within the framework of preoperative clarification, when the operating surgeon sets out trying to draw up a plan for curative surgery and is surprised by an advanced tumor. Choosing the correct procedure in situations such as this always carries a heavy burden. The great responsibility of the operating surgeon is best borne when based on a trusting relationship with the patient.

Another task in cases of incurable or inoperable patients, which to a large extent still awaits adequate resolution, is encountered in the postoperative phase. Neither retreating to analgesics nor clouding the situation can meet the needs of tumor patients. It is precisely in the patient who has undergone palliative surgery that a gross distortion of his condition will result in a loss of trust and in bitterness. All too often, the patient feels isolated and alone in the unavoidable crisis which he is in. Gently explaining the real situation to the patient can provide a renewed basis for hope, even if only for a short time.

References

1. Schreiber HW, Eichfuss HP, Kortmann KB: Palliativeingriffe an Speiseröhre und Magen. Chirurg 1981;52:1.
2. Cook AO, Levine BA, Sirinek KR, et al: Evaluation of gastric adenocarcinoma. Abdominal computed tomography does not replace celiotomy. Arch Surg 1986; 121:603.
3. Tio TL, Den Härtog Jager FCA, et al: The role of endoscopic ultrasonography in assessing local resectability of oesophagogastric malignancies. Scand J Gastroenterol 1986;21(suppl 12):78.
4. Madden MV, Price SK, Learmonth GM, et al: Surgical staging of gastric carcinoma: sources and consequences of error. Br J Surg 1987;74:119.
5. Cunningham D, Hole D, Taggart DJ, et al: Evaluation of the prognostic factors in gastric cancer: the effect of chemotherapy on survival. Br J Surg 1987;74:715.
6. Kirchner R, Henke W, Wittekind C, et al: The surgeon's estimation of radicality and results of pathologic examination at margins of resection in gastric cancer surgery. Scand J Gastroenterol 1987;22(suppl 133):72.
7. Siewert JR, Lange J, Böttcher K, et al: Magenkarzinom-Bestandsaufnahme aus chirurgischer Sicht. Dtsch Med Wschr 1987;112:622.
8. Srivastav A, Hughes LE: Role of palliative surgery in gastric cancer, in Preece PE, Cuschieri A, Wellwood JM (eds): Cancer of the Stomach. Orlando, Grune & Stratton, 1986, p. 189.

9. British Stomach Cancer Group: Resection line disease in stomach cancer. Br Med J 1984;289:601.
10. Ekbom GA, Gleysteen JJ: Gastric malignancy: resection for palliation. Surgery 1980;884:476.
11. Herfarth C, Schreiber HW: Palliativeingriffe beim nichtresektions-fähigen Magenkarzinom, in Becker HD, Lierse W, Schreiber HW (eds): Magenchirurgie. Berlin-Heidelberg-New York, Springer, 1986, p. 160.
12. Junginger T, Muschong N, Pichlmaier H: Palliative Verfahren bei Magenkarzinom. Münch Med Wschr 1984;126:440.
13. Stern JL, Denman S, Elias NY, et al: Evaluation of palliative resection in advanced carcinoma of the stomach. Surgery 1975;77:291.
14. Niederle B, Roka R, Schemper M, et al: Bypassoperationen beim nichtresezierbaren Ösophagus-Kardia-Karzinom. Akt Chir 1986;21:104.
15. Feifel G, Hildebrandt U, Koch B: Tumorbedingte gastrointestinale Perforation: chirurgische Therapie. Münch Med Wschr 1987;129:262.
16. Maruyama K: The most important prognostic factors for gastric cancer patients. A study using univariate and multivariate analyses. Scand J Gastroenterol 1987;22(suppl 133):63.
17. Buchholtz TW, Welch CE, Malt RA: Clinical correlates of resectability and survival in gastric carcinoma. Ann Surg 1978;6:711.
18. Koga S, Kawaguchi H, Kishimoto H, et al: Therapeutic significance of noncurative gastrectomy for gastric cancer with liver metastasis. Amer J Surg 1980;140:356.
19. Moertel CG: The natural history of advanced gastric cancer. Surg Gynecol Obstet 1968;126:1071.
20. Beckmann J, Ditlev G, Blichert-Toft M, in Aaranson N, Beckmann J (eds): The Quality of Life in Cancer Patients. New York, Raven Press, 1987.

CHAPTER 8

The Surgical Treatment of Carcinoma in the Operated Stomach

P. Langhans and G. Heidl

Introduction

In the more than100-year history of gastric surgery, an enormous number of clinical and experimental studies laid the groundwork for the effective surgical treatment of ulcers in practice today. Despite this, all surgical procedures continue to have undesirable side effects. These may take the form of early and late complications with a considerable number of symptoms and signs; they may cause general insufficiencies; or they may bring about slowly progressing chronic changes in gastric morphology. While the results of gastric surgery and the early consequences of ulcer surgery remain clear to the individual surgeon and gastroenterologist, no one reckoned with the most dangerous and insidious late complication associated with the latter–carcinoma in the operated stomach. This tumor develops only after an average postoperative interval of 25 years and therefore easily eludes individual detection.[1]

Definition

The following conditions must be met in order to distinguish carcinoma of the gastric stump from other gastric carcinomas:

1. In the case of a benign indication for surgery, an interval of at least 5 years prior to the second illness is required for reliable elimination of misdiagnoses.
2. In the case of a malignant indication for surgery, an interval of 20 years is required to ensure permanent recovery from the primary illness up to the onset of a second malignancy.
3. In the case of a first operation, morphologic changes in the gastric wall along the lines of scar tissue formation or continuous disruptions in gastric physiology must be present.

Based on our experimental and clinical results, we coined the term "gastric carcinoma resulting from surgery" for this lesion, which comes about following operations on carcinoma-free stomachs.[2,3]

Our Patients

From 1973 to 1987, 113 patients with gastric carcinoma resulting from surgery were treated at the Surgical University Hospital in Münster. Using the aforementioned definition, six patients had their ulcers treated as the first operation, six underwent a simple gastroenterostomy, four a Billroth I resection, and 97 a Billroth II resection (the retrocolic gastroenterostomy modification in 82 and the anterocolic gastroenterostomy modification in the remaining 15) (Fig. 1). The average free interval measured 25 years in our patients, which was in accordance with the length of the free interval between surgical procedures for a benign condition up to the appearance of a carcinoma in the resected stomach cited in published literature. The variations ranged between 10 and 50 years.

Given the generally advanced age of the patients with carcinoma of the gastric stump (mean of 65 years in our patients) and the anticipated major surgical intervention, the decision to proceed with a radical method is often not easily made during the evaluation of operability. At the most, a residual gastrectomy can satisfy the requirement for curability in the case of carcinoma of the gastric stump if one were to try and do justice to the basic principle of tumor surgery of the gastrointestinal tract: resection of the diseased tissue with subsequent anatomical and function-dependent reconstruction. The surgeon is often forced to perform operations that do not place too much strain on the patient—to the disadvantage of radical surgery—but which benefit the patient's remaining quality of life.

From the standpoint of treatment, curative surgery was possible in 45.1% of all of our patients, with the possibility of palliative resection or gastrectomy in 16.8%. A total of 32.8% of all operations were concluded by exploratory laparotomy, and quality of life was improved by endotubation. Surgery was not performed in 5.3% of the patients because of absolute inoperability (Fig. 2). Only 21% of patients who underwent radical surgery are still alive today, although most have not yet reached the 5-year recovery limit. Nevertheless, nine early carcinomas with a known more favorable prognosis are included in this statistic. The data obtained in our patients, together with those reported in published

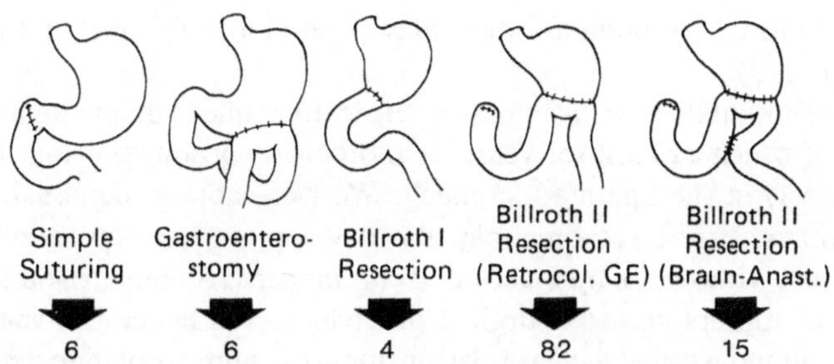

Fig. 1. Incidence of carcinomas in the resected stomach after various surgical procedures. Patients at the Surgical University Hospital, Münster, 1973–1987.

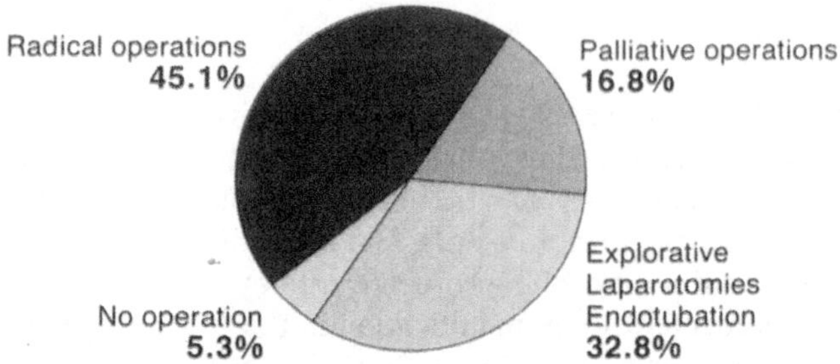

Fig. 2. Treatment during carcinoma in the resected stomach. Patients at the Surgical University Hospital, Münster, 1973–1987.

literature, underscore the poor prognosis of this carcinoma. Preventive medical examinations and prophylactic surgical measures are therefore necessary to uncover precancerous stages or at least carcinomas in an early stage and possibly to prevent development using suitable surgical procedures.

Predisposing Factors

Of the numerous factors predisposing to carcinoma of the gastric stump, those of primary concern are nonphysiologically elevated duodenogastric reflux, chronic atrophic gastritis, scar formation on the anastomosis, two different kinds of adjoining epithelia, differing suture materials, lysolecithin as an agent damaging to the mucosal barrier, bacterially induced N-nitrosation in the stomach, induced hypochlorhydria, and, more recently, immunological factors (Table 1).

While causality has yet to be proven for the majority of these strongly suspected factors, bacterially induced nitrosation and duodenogastric reflux have been examined experimentally and clinically. Schlag and co-workers[4,5] showed that changes in the acidity ratios alter intragastric bacterial colonization. They concluded from the qualitative and quantitative changes in the intragastric bacterial flora that direct bacterial cytotoxicity, bacterial metabolic activity in bile-acid metabolism, and the reduction of nitrate to nitrite as well as its capacity to catalyze *N*-nitroso compounds may play a carcinogenic role in the operated stomach (Fig. 3).

Increased stimulation resulting from surgically induced duodenogastric reflux, the effect of which can last for years, is another important contributing factor to carcinogenesis in the operated stomach. We were able to demonstrate experimentally that gastric carcinoma may also develop after an equivalent biological interval, even without the application of carcinogens. A comparison between the incidence of tumors and the surgical procedure, and hence the varying reflux intensities, demonstrated a clear relationship—the number of detected malignant growths increased considerably as a function of the intensity of the duodenogastric reflux. The carcinomas discovered in the experiments appear only after

Table 1. Predisposing factors for cancer in the resected stomach

Predisposing factor	Reference
Scarring at the anastomosis	Beatson GT: Carcinoma of the stomach after gastrojejunostomy. Br Med J 1926;I:15.
Mechanical irritation of the wound	Angerer H: Zur Histologie alter Gastroenterostomiestellen und deren Umgebung. Dtsch Z Chir 1927;201:229.
Disturbance of mucosal blood supply	Lurje A: Krebs der gastroenteroanastomotischen Öffnung. Zentrabl Chir 1935;62:2304.
Chronic atrophic gastritis	Konjetzny GE: Der Magenkrebs. Stuttgart, Enke, 1938.
Chemical irritation by alkaline intestinal contents	Beyer W: Zur Frage des Gastroenterostomiekrebses und seiner örtlichen Vorbedingungen. Arch Klin Chir 1943;204:445.
Induced hypochlorhydria	Debray C, Roux M, Chevillotte R, et al: Les cancers due moignon gastrique après gastrectomie pour ulcus. Arch Mal App Dig 1950;39:702.
Joining of two different types of intestinal mucosa	Becker T, Freund E: Magenkarzinom und Ulcuschirurgie. Zentralbl Chir 1964;89:455.
Destruction of mucosal barrier by lysolecithin	Davenport HW: Effect of lysolecithine, digitonin, and phospholipase upon the gastric mucosal barrier. Gastroenterology 1970;59:505.
Intragastric nitrosation	Schlag P, Meister H, Feyerabend G, et al: Der Einfluss des duodenogastrischen Refluxes auf das Epithel an der gastroenteralen Anastomose. Langenbecks Arch Klin Chir 1977;344:207.
Residual suture material	Schönleben K, Langhans P, Schlake W, et al: Gastric stump carcinoma–cancerogenic factors and possible preventive measures. Acta Hepatogastroenterol 1979;26:239.
Immunologic factors	Reissigl H, Schwamberger K: Der operierte Magen–eine Präkanzerose? in Beger HG, Bergemann W, Oshima H (eds): Das Magenkarzinom–Frühdiagnose und Therapie. Stuttgart-New York, Thieme, 1980, p. 38.
Reflux-induced cellular proliferation	Langhans P, Bues M, Heger RA, et al: Zellkinetische Untersuchungen mit ^{3}H-Thymidin im operierten Rattenmagen. Z Gastroenterol 1982;20:574.

certain changes in gastric physiology and may be avoided entirely, given the appropriate surgical procedure. Since these carcinomas are caused only by surgical procedures in animals not afflicted with any preliminary illnesses or gastric cancer, to describe carcinoma in the operated stomach as "carcinoma resulting from surgery" would appear justified.

The Billroth II resection with gastroenterostomy according to Roux has been proven experimentally to be an effective operative procedure. Malignant growths do not appear to be associated with this modification, in which the reflux remains within physiological limits. With all due precaution regarding the extrapolation of experimental animal results to humans, we may conclude that for the surgical prophylaxis of carcinoma resulting from surgery, those procedures that prevent reflux are probably preferable (Figs. 4 and 5).[2,6]

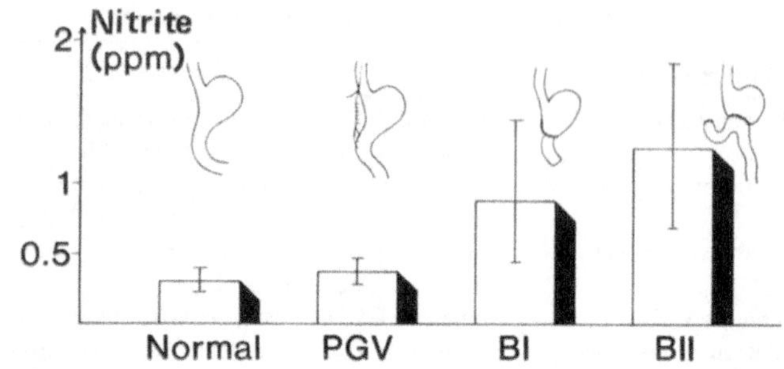

Fig. 3. Intragastric nitrite concentration given normal individuals and various types of gastric surgery. (Modification according to Schlag P, Böckler R, Ulrich H, et al: Are nitrite and N-nitroso compounds in gastric juice risk factors for carcinoma in the operated stomach? *Lancet* 1980;1:727).

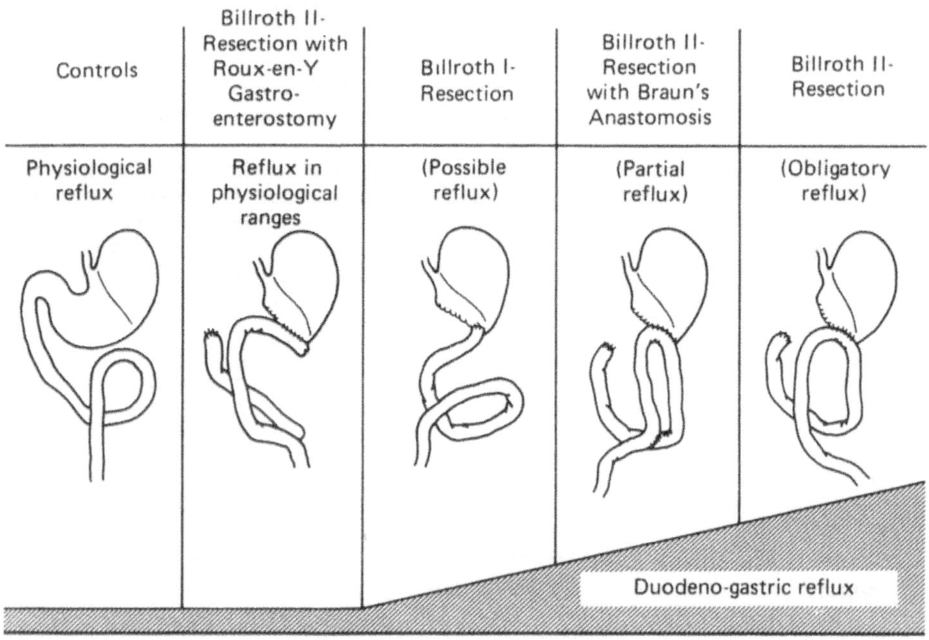

Fig. 4. Reflux ratios following various resectional surgical procedures in animal experiments.

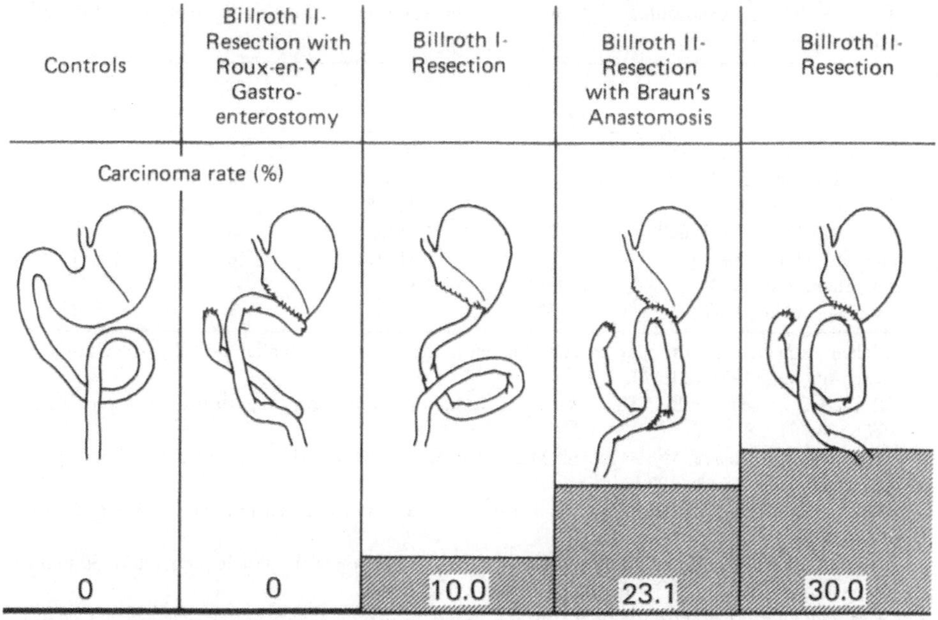

Fig. 5. Incidence of carcinoma (%) in a stomach following resectional surgical procedures in animal experiments.

Postoperative Free Interval

Although the gastric stump is recognized as a "precancerous condition," the value of preventive medical examinations continues to be questioned because the associated cancer risk is underestimated. The average free interval of 25 years in our patients was in agreement with the length of the free interval between surgical procedures from a benign condition to the appearance of a carcinoma in the resected stomach as cited in the literature. The variations measured between 10 and 15 years. Retrospective follow-ups from the literature which take a postoperative interval of that length into account clearly show that the gastric stump is associated with an elevated risk of cancer (Table 2). Authors who arrive at these risk assessments based on much shorter periods of observation may rightly be accused of lacking the necessary experience about this topic. One could otherwise not conclude that the incidence of cancer in the gastric stump rises significantly in comparison to that of an intact stomach only after a 17-year postoperative interval, as Domellöf and Janunger[7] calculated in an extensive 1977 study (Fig. 6). It is precisely this fact, however, which most authors who view the risk of cancer in the resected stomach as slight overlook.

Table 2. The assessment of cancer risk in the resected stomach according to published follow-up studies

Authors	Follow-up cases (n)	Interval (years)	Cancer incidence	Estimated risk
Helsingen, Hillestad 1956[a]	220	10–35	11	↑
Domellöf, Janunger 1977[b]	676	>12	14	↑
Schrumpf, et al 1977[c]	421	20–25	7	↑
Welvaart, Warnsinck 1982[d]	264	>26	5	↔
Pickford, et al 1984[e]	632	31–39	18	↑
v de Stadt, et al 1984[f]	1245	15–44	48	↑
Langhans, et al 1985[g]	330	5–45	7	↑

[a] Helsingen N, Hillestad L: Cancer development in the gastric stump after partial gastrectomy for ulcer. Ann Surg 1956;143:173.

[b] Domellöf L, Janungen KG: The risk for gastric carcinoma after partial gastrectomy. Amer J Surg 1977;134:581.

[c] Schrumpf E, Stadaas J, Myren J, et al: Mucosal changes in the gastric stump 20–25 years after partial gastrectomy. Lancet 1977;2:467.

[d] Welvaart K, Warnsinck HM: The incidence of carcinoma of the gastric remnant. J Surg Oncol 1982;21:104.

[e] Pickford IR, Craven JL, Hall R, et al: Endoscopic examination of the gastric remnant 31–39 years after subtotal gastrectomy for peptic ulcer. Gut 1984;25:393.

[f] v de Stadt J, Offerhaus GJA, de Boer J, et al: Carcinoom en premaligne veranderingen in biopten uit de maag ven patiënten die mer dan 15 yaar geleden een maagoperatie ondergingen. Ned Tÿdschr Geneeskd 1984;128:606.

[g] Langhans P, Böttcher K, Bünte H: Das Krebsproblem des operierten Magens – Präkanzerosen als Indikation zum Korrektureingriff, in Bünte H, Langhans P, Meyer HJ, et al (eds): Aktuelle Therapie des Magenkarzinoms. Berlin-Heidelberg-New York, Springer, 1985, p 143.

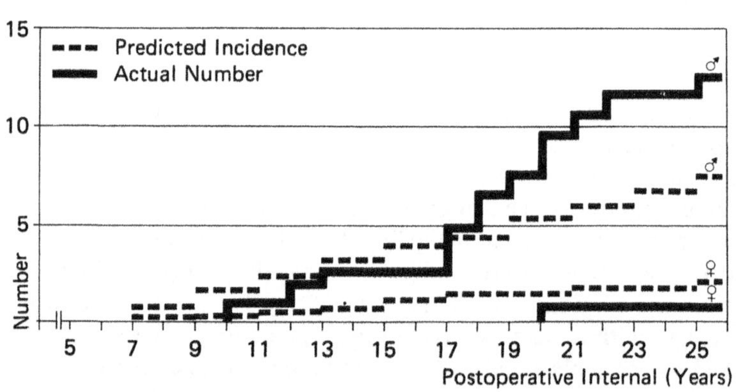

Fig. 6. Expected and actual incidence of carcinoma in the resected stomach (modification according to Domellöf L, Janunger KG: The risk for gastric carcinoma after partial gastrectomy. *Amer J Surg* 1977;134:581).

Surgical Procedure and Cancer Risk

Another aspect of the assessment of cancer risk concerns the previous surgical procedure. Since carcinomas are at present primarily observed following Billroth II resections, the inevitable question is: Which surgical procedure entails the highest or lowest risk?

The incidence of carcinoma following Billroth II resections observed in our patients also should not be taken as an absolute value but should be considered in light of the history of ulcer surgery. As shown graphically in Figure 7, the number of simple gastroenterostomies performed reached a peak in 1920, with the most Billroth II resections performed in 1960. The Billroth I resection became accepted as a routine procedure only after the 1960s, and vagotomy is currently at its peak.

Carcinogenesis following simple gastroenterostomy peaked in 1945, and this procedure has not been performed routinely for many years. Consequently, few carcinomas resulting from simple gastroenterostomy are seen today, whereas a large number of gastric stump carcinomas following Billroth II resections can be observed. The incidence of carcinomas following Billroth I resections is expected to peak around the year 2005.

It therefore goes without saying that assessing the risk of cancer following vagotomy is impossible at the present time (Fig. 7). But the presumed slight or

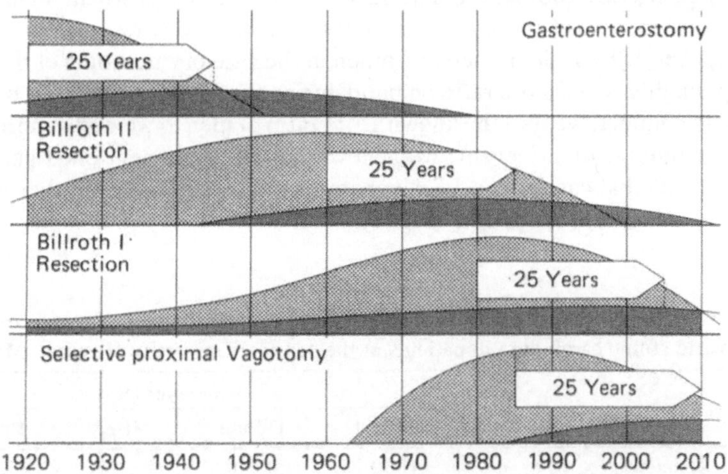

Fig. 7. Expected incidence peak of carcinomas in a resected stomach as a function of the previous surgical procedure taking into account the history of ulcer surgery (modification according to Heger RA, Langhans P, Hohenstein J: Risikoeinschätzung von Spätkomplikationen in der Ulkuschirurgie, in Bünte H, Langhans P (eds): *100 Jahre Ulkus-Chirurgie.* Munich-Vienna-Baltimore, Urban & Schwarzenberg, 1982, p. 282).

absent cancer risk presented as an argument for vagotomy should not encourage its use as long as no comparative long-term results with the resection procedure exist.[6,8] We therefore cannot say with certainty which surgical procedure results in the highest cancer burden.

Morphological Differences: Gastric Carcinoma – Carcinoma of the Gastric Stump

In light of the synopses of experimental and clinical studies as well as pathological and histological findings, the gastric stump must be viewed today as a "precancerous condition" entailing a considerable risk of cancer. The retrospective evaluation of all carcinomas of the 101 tumors following first resections and the Laurén classification also indicate that a varying cancer risk does indeed exist in the gastric stump, independent of surgical procedure.[9] We were able to determine that the ratio of intestinal to diffuse types of carcinoma compared with carcinoma of the gastric stump measures 1.46:1, compared with normal gastric carcinoma, with a ratio of 0.92:1 (Table 3). Assuming the normal gastric carcinoma to have endogenic and exogenic components, the higher rate of the intestinal type in carcinomas of the operated stomach is to be viewed as an index for the development of this carcinoma, which results, among other factors, from the exogenic stimulation or the chronic stimulation of the duodenogastric reflux. This ratio also agrees with published data on this subject. While only a handful of authors have shed any light on this problem and compared types of tumors with normal gastric carcinoma, the data seem to confirm our postulate (Table 4).

The distribution of the two carcinomas between the sexes also varies enormously. The 5.7:1 ratio of men to women in the case of carcinoma of the gastric stump roughly reflects the ratio on hand during the initial surgery (ie, ulcer surgery). In contrast, we find the known 1.4:1 ratio of men to women in normal gastric carcinomas. In any event, we believe that the aforementioned parameters also indicate that carcinomas of the operated stomach involve another independent type of gastric carcinoma (Fig. 8).

Table 3. Classification of tumor type according to Laurén in cases of gastric carcinoma and gastric stump carcinoma in patients at the surgical University Hospital, Münster

	Tumor type (%)			
	Intestinal	Diffuse	Mixed	Unclassified
Gastric carcinoma (n = 306)	41.72	45.70	6.90	2.98
	0.92:1			
Carcinoma of the gastric stump (n = 101)	50.50	34.70	13.90	.90
	1.46:1			

Table 4. Classification of carcinoma in an operated stomach, according to Laurén: Review of the literature

Authors	No. cases	Type, per Laurén		
		Intestinal	Diffuse	Other
Taksdal, Stalsberg 1973[a]	84	38 (45.2%)	33 (39.3%)	13 (15.5%)
Hammar 1976[b]	56	27 (48.2%)	29 (51.8%)	–
Hermanek, Riemann 1982[c]	94	38 (40.0%)	?	?
Schwamberger 1983[d]	279	146 (52.3%)	70 (25.0%)	63 (22.7%)
Pickford, et al 1984[e]	9	8 (88.9%)	1 (11.1%)	–

[a] Taksdal S, Stalsberg H: Histology of gastric carcinoma occurring after gastric surgery for benign condition. Cancer 1973;32:162.

[b] Hammar E: The localization of precancerous changes and carcinoma after previous gastric operation for benign condition. Acta Path Microbiol Scand 1976;84 (section A):495.

[c] Hermanek P, Riemann JF: The operated stomach–still a precancerous condition? (editorial). Endoscopy 1982;14:113.

[d] Schwamberger K: Magenstumpfkarzinom: pathogenese und therapie, in Demling L, Lux G, Domschke W (eds): Therapie postoperativer Störungen des Gastrointestinaltraktes. Stuttgart-New York, Thieme, 1983, p 185.

[e] Pickford IR, Craven JL, Hall R, et al: Endoscopic examination of the gastric remnant 31–39 years after subtotal gastrectomy for peptic ulcer. Gut 1984;25:393.

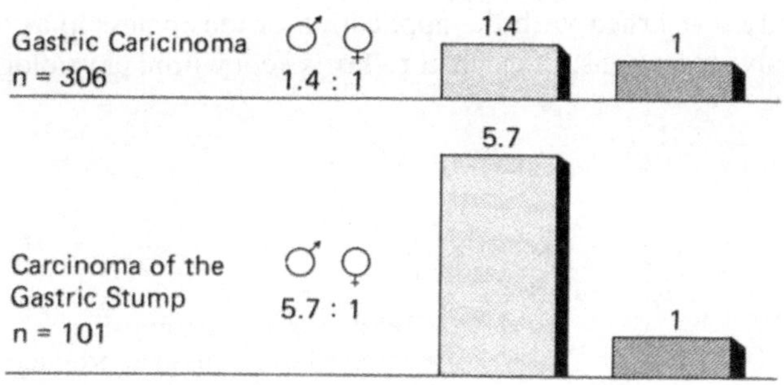

Fig. 8. Sex ratios of patients with gastric carcinoma and gastric-stump carcinoma (Surgical University Hospital, Münster).

Postulates for Practice

Even if the interrelationships between surgery and the later development of carcinoma have been proven on the basis of clinical and experimental studies, some of the causes of this multifactorial cancer phenomenon remain hypothetical. In terms of carcinogenesis, the nonphysiologically elevated influx of bile and pancreatic juices is probably the most important causal factor. Until proven different, however, the surgeon's goal must be to carry out prophylactic operations that prevent reflux by drawing upon improved surgical procedures. The gastroenterologist must be able to recognize this secondary disease in its early or most risky stage within the framework of systematic preventive examinations of the patient or for diagnostic purposes, for a therapeutically curative surgical intervention, or for a corrective operation in a reflux-free procedure at the right time.

Surgical Prophylaxis

With the idea that gastric reflux can be prevented by means of a Roux loop following gastric resection with reconstruction of the gastrointestinal tract, in the early 1970s we reintroduced the technique inaugurated by Roux in 1893.[10,11] In addition to the advantages relating to surgical technique, which in this method are primarily concerned with the application of tensionless anastomoses, even after extensive resections, the jejunal reflux is kept within physiological limits by

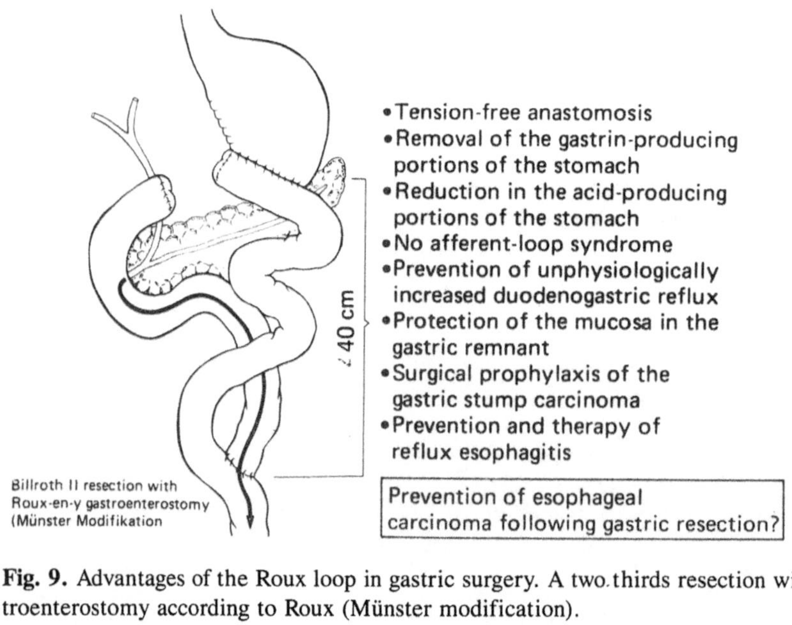

Fig. 9. Advantages of the Roux loop in gastric surgery. A two thirds resection with gastroenterostomy according to Roux (Münster modification).

means of a sufficiently long Roux loop. Secondary diseases such as reflux gastritis or reflux esophagitis either no longer occur after this modification or are surgically treated via transformation in this procedure (Fig. 9).

We can only hope that the reflux-free resection procedure represents the desired advance for resective ulcer surgery and can actually prevent the gastric carcinoma resulting from surgery. Nearly 15 years' experience with this resection procedure permits us, based on pathomorphologic considerations among others, to continue to favor this reflux-reducing surgical procedure for ulcer surgery.[3,10]

Preventive Medical Examination of Gastric Surgery Patients

Precisely because of the different answers to the question concerning the reversibility of dysplasias, as well as to the resultant clinical and therapeutic consequences, individuals having undergone gastric surgery must be included in a strict postoperative care program (Fig. 10). At our clinic, all gastric surgical patients are therefore invited to our "gastroenterologic consulting hour" for a first follow-up examination at the latest 15 years after ulcer surgery. All examinations suited for recognizing postoperative syndromes and morphological changes

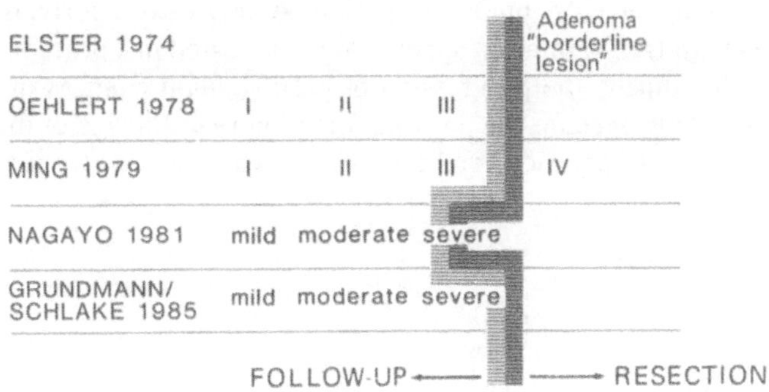

Fig. 10. The evaluation of dysplasias in the resected stomach by several pathologists: follow-up or resection.

[a]Elster K: Doubtful cases and precancerous lesions (indicative list of various methods), in Grundmann E, Grunze H, Witte S (eds): *Early Gastric Cancer.* Berlin-Heidelberg-New York, Springer, 1974, p. 176.

[b]Oehlert W: *Klinische Pathologie des Magen-Darm-Traktes.* Stuttgart-New York, Schattauer, 1978.

[c]Ming SC: Dysplasia of the gastric epithelium. *Front Gastrointest Res* 1979;4:164.

[d]Nagayo T: Histological diagnosis of biopsied gastric mucosa with special reference to that of borderline lesions. *Gann* 1971;11:245.

[e]Grundmann E, Schlake W: Präkanzeröse Läsionen der Magenschleimhaut, in Bünte H, Langhans P, Meyer HJ, et al (eds): *Aktuelle Therapie des Magenkarzinoms.* Berlin-Heidelberg-New York, Springer, 1985, p. 15.

Table 5. The importance of endoscopy for the prevention of carcinoma in the resected stomach

Exact morphologic diagnosis
Follow-up examinations at optimal intervals
Detection of progressive mucosal changes
Early detection of gastric carcinoma in the operated stomach
Improving prognosis

in the stomach are performed at the precancerous stage, at least in the early stage of cancer. Of particular importance in this regard is endoscopy in conjunction with biopsy, which enables a precise morphological diagnosis with a check of the findings at prudent intervals, the recognition of the progression of a gastric carcinoma, and the early detection of a gastric carcinoma with a considerable improvement in prognosis (Table 5).

The follow-up examination intervals are kept flexible from the outset and are set again on an individual basis after each examination. In the case of a severe dysplasia established via biopsy and histology, the patient should be checked at the end of 6 months. In cases of mild chronic changes in the gastric mucosa, an examination after 5 years is generally sufficient. If and when a preventive second operation should be carried out—even when premalignant change in the gastric mucosa exists—is currently under discussion. At any rate, a corrective surgical intervention with transformation appears to be indicated in a procedure less burdened by reflux during the progression of premalignant changes in the gastric mucosa, taking into account the postoperative interval, the age of the patient at the time of the first operation, and the disease which led to the first operation (Table 6).[12,13]

Summary

The prognosis for carcinoma in an operated stomach is exceptionally poor because the diagnosis is in most cases made too late. In light of the high cancer risk of former gastric surgical patients, preventive measures are indicated. Follow-up examinations should be arranged at appropriate intervals for the individual patient. Assuming that preventive medical examinations can spare some patients of cancer, we feel compelled to continue to adhere to our postulate for a prevention program. The diagnosis for resection procedures in ulcer surgery should be made sparingly. Should a resection be indicated, reflux-reducing anastomotic techniques should be drawn upon in each case. Corrective surgery with transformation in a procedure less burdened by reflux appears to be indicated during the progression of premalignant changes in the stomach and mucosa taking into account the postoperative interval, the age of the patient at the time of the first operation, and the disease that led to the first operation.

Table 6. Factors that help determine the indication for corrective surgery in the resected stomach

Progressive development of premalignant changes in the gastric mucosa
Duration of the postoperative interval
Age of the patient at first operation
Basic disease demanding first surgical intervention
Onset or increase of complaints
Onset of functional disorders

References

1. Heger RA, Langhans P, Hohenstein J: Risikoeinschätzung von Spätkomplikationen in der Ulkuschirurgie, in Bünte H, Langhans P (eds): 100 Jahre Ulkus-Chirurgie. Munich-Vienna-Baltimore, Urban & Schwarzenberg, 1982, p. 282.
2. Langhans P, Heger RA, Hohenstein J, et al: Das Operationsfolgekarzinom des Magens – eine experimentelle Studie. Therapiewoche 1980;30:8475.
3. Langhans P: Die Roux-Schlinge in der Ulkuschirurgie, in Bünte H, Grill W, Langhans P, et al (eds): Die Roux-Schlinge, Indikationen, Techniken und Resultate. Edition Medizin. Deerfield Beach-Basel, Weinheim, 1984, p. 151.
4. Schlag P, Meister H, Feyerabend G, et al: Der Einfluss des duodenogastrischen Refluxes auf das Epithel an der gastroenteralen Anastomose. Langenbecks Arch Klin Chir 1977;344:207.
5. Schlag P, Böckler R, Ulrich H, et al: Are nitrite and N-nitroso compounds in gastric juice risk factors for carcinoma in the operated stomach? Lancet 1980;1:727.
6. Langhans P, Heger RA, Stegemann B: The cancer risk in the stomach subjected to nonresecting procedure – an experimental long-term study. Scand J Gastroenterol 1984;19 (suppl 92):138.
7. Domellöf L, Janunger KG: The risk for gastric carcinoma after partial gastrectomy. Amer J Surg 1977;134:581.
8. Langhans P: Das Krebsrisiko des operierten Magens – eine Standortbestimmung, in Häring R: Therapie des Magenkarzinoms. Edition Medizin. Deerfield Beach-Basel, Weinheim, 1984, p. 31.
9. Laurén P: The two histological main types of gastric carcinoma: diffuse and so-called intestinal-type carcinoma. Acta Path Microbiol Scand 1965;64:31.
10. Langhans P, Schönleben K, Bünte H: The routine use of Roux-en-Y anastomosis in gastric surgery. Scand J Gastroenterol 1981;16(suppl 67):247.
11. Roux C: De la gastroenterostomie. Etude, basée sur les opérations pratiqués du 21. Juin 1888 au 1 Septembre 1896. Rev Gynecol Chir Abdominale 1897;1:67.
12. Langhans P, Bues M, Heger RA: When is a corrective procedure indicated for the operated stomach? Scand J Gastroenterol 1984;19 (suppl 92):235.
13. Langhans P, Böttcher K, Bünte H: Das Krebsproblem des operierten Magens – Präkanzerosen als Indikation zum Korrektureingriff, in Bünte H, Langhans P, Meyer HJ, et al (eds): Aktuelle Therapie des Magenkarzinoms. Berlin-Heidelberg-New York, Springer, 1985, p. 143.

CHAPTER 9

Follow-Up Care and Surgery for Recurrent Gastric Cancer

P. Schlag, K. Buhl, and C. Herfarth

Introduction

Despite potentially curative surgery, the incidence of recurrence of gastric carcinoma is relatively high. In addition to tumor aggressiveness and growth characteristics, surgical strategy is a determining factor in the frequency of recurrence.[1-3] Recurrence can take the form of distant metastases or peritoneal carcinomatosis, hence reflecting disseminated tumor disease. At present no cure is possible in this situation. The degree to which cytostatic treatment, given an early diagnosis of metastases, leads to improved prognosis and whether cure may be achieved through renewed surgical treatment, given localized tumor recurrence, are unresolved issues. This is presumed in the requirement for routine follow-up care of gastric cancer patients following partial or total gastrectomy.[4,5]

Although up to 90% of all recurrences are expected within the first 2 years following surgery,[1,6] recurrence can take place several years later as well.[7] Regional recurrence (anastomosis, epigastric lymph nodes) must be distinguished from generalized tumor metastases (peritoneal carcinomatosis, organ metastases). Recurrences are most often encountered in the gastric remnant, so that their differentiation from metachronic second carcinoma is frequently difficult. The frequency of follow-up care and course of examinations must be oriented to the known progression of recurrence over time and focused at the most likely sites of recurrence.

The standardization of follow-up care attainable in this way, coupled with the simultaneous application of increasingly sensitive examination techniques, including the serial determination of so-called tumor markers (CEA, Ca 19-9), should contribute to the early diagnosis of recurrence and hence to the desired improved prognosis.[8-10] The extent to which this may be realized will be analyzed subsequently in greater detail based on our experience.

Patients and Methods

A total of 372 patients with gastric carcinoma were treated surgically at our Surgical Department from October 1, 1983 to October 1, 1986 (Fig. 1). Tumor could

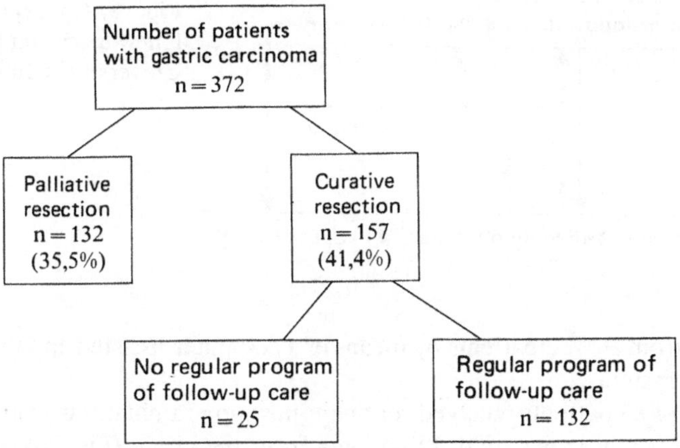

Fig. 1. Follow-up care for gastric carcinoma.

be resected in 77% of the patients, with the objective of cure in 157 patients. All but 25 of the patients who had undergone curative operations received routine follow-up examinations according to the protocol outlined in Figure 2. Patients as well as their respective family physicians received timely reminders from the tumor registry about upcoming follow-up examinations. The patients could choose to have the follow-up care examinations carried out primarily by the family physician, if necessary with the participation of specialist resident physicians, or directly during the office hours arranged for follow-up care at our clinic (Fig. 3). Feedback of results from the examinations to the tumor registry was

		Postop. month following radical first operation													
		2	4	6	8	10	12	15	18	21	24	30	36	42	48
Base Program	Physical exam CEA BSG, HB, GPT, AP, γ-GT	●	●	●	●	●	●	●	●	●	●	●	●	●	●
Special program 1. Gastrectomy 2. Gastric resection or gastrectomy given proximal tumor	Endoscopy	●		●		●		●			●				●
Additional program	Epigastric sonograph			●			●		●		●		●		●
	Thoracic X-ray						●				●		●		●
	GI series			●											

Fig. 2. Follow-up care program for patients with gastric carcinoma.

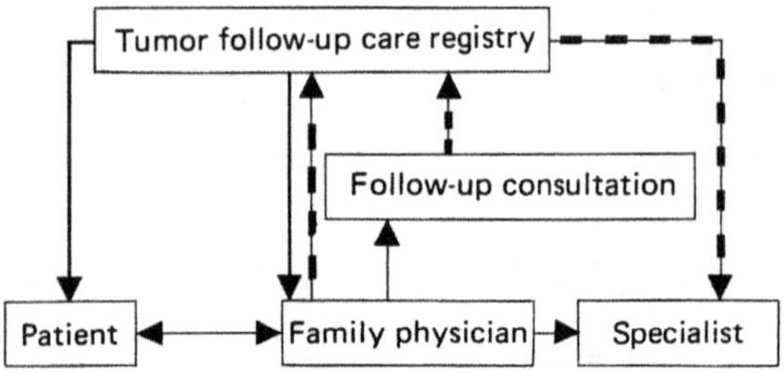

Fig. 3. Concept of tumor follow-up care at the Surgical University Clinic, Heidelberg.

obtained from all 132 patients by means of a computer-assisted appointment and reminder system.

A total of 83 patients received routine follow-up examinations primarily from their family physicians, and 49 patients from the clinic (Fig. 4A). Minimum duration of follow-up was 1 year, with an average duration of 32 months.

Results

Tumor recurrence has been diagnosed in 33 patients to date. The higher proportion of recurrence discovered in patients followed up at the clinic may be explained by their more advanced stage of primary tumor (Table 1). Indepen-

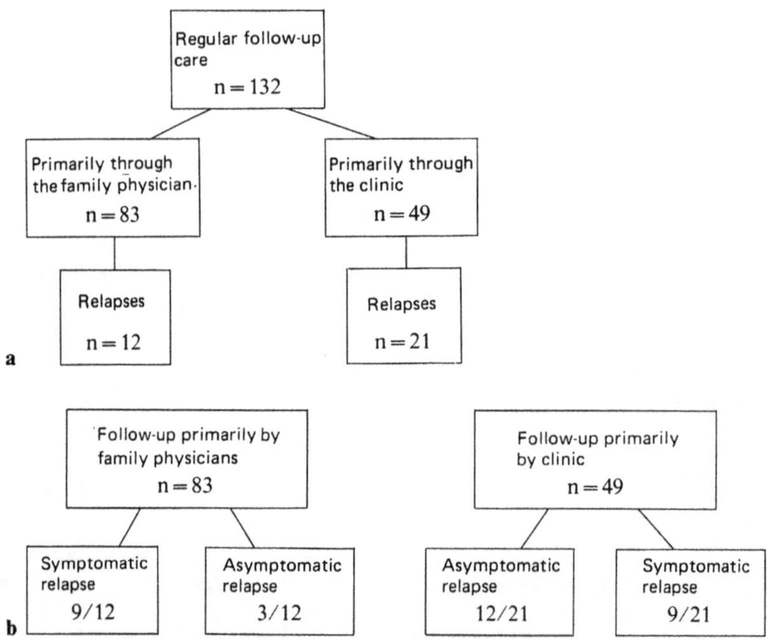

Fig. 4. (**a**) Follow-up care for gastric carcinoma. (**b**) Follow-up care for gastric carcinoma.

Table 1. Follow-up care for gastric carcinoma

	Primary tumor		
	Stage I	Stage II	Stage III
Follow-up primarily by family physician	53%	20%	27%
Follow-up primarily by clinic	17%	31%	52%

dently, tumor recurrence was detected mostly in asymptomatic patients within the framework of the follow-up examinations at the clinic (Fig. 4B). Metastases to the liver and lung, which were largely detectable by sonography or x-rays, predominated in asymptomatic patients (Table 2). In contrast, peritoneal carcinomatosis often remained undetected within the framework of follow-up care until the appearance of clinical symptoms.

Seven of the 33 patients with recurrent tumor were operated on a second time (Table 3). In symptomatic patients, reoperation was performed in part because of emergency situations due to ileus caused by peritoneal dissemination. Resection of tumor was not possible in any of these patients. Surprisingly, a greater proportion of asymptomatic patients with recurrent tumor could undergo systemic chemotherapy than could symptomatic patients. The possibility of early secondary treatment had only an apparent advantage with respect to the survival time (Table 4). While the median survival time of the asymptomatic patients was twice that of the symptomatic patients following the diagnosis of recurrence, the overall survival times of the two groups, as measured from the time of primary treatment, did not differ.

Discussion

Our results are essentially in agreement with earlier experiences of follow-up care of gastric carcinoma patients subjected to potentially curative operations.[8,11-14] While it was possible to record a comparatively high proportion of asymptomatic recurrences by means of the standardized and highly involved follow-up examination program,[13,14] this did not lead to the expected therapeutic

Table 2. Follow-up care for gastric cancer: Influence on recurrence pattern

	Local recurrence	Peritoneal carcinomatosis (seedings)	Distant metastases
Asymptomatic patients	2/15 (13%)	3/15 (20%)	10/15 (67%)
Symptomatic patients	2/18 (11%)	13/18 (72%)	3/18 (17%)

Surgical University Clinic, Heidelberg.

Table 3. Follow-up care of gastric cancer: Therapeutic procedures during detection of recurrence

Asymptomatic patients			Symptomatic patients		
Chemotherapy	Surgery	No specific therapy	Chemotherapy	Surgery	No specific therapy
8/15 (53%)	1/15 (7%)	5/15 (33%)	2/18 (11%)	6/18 (33%)	10/18 (55%)

Surgical University Clinic, Heidelberg.

Table 4. Survival times of patients with recurrence of gastric carcinoma

	Median survival time after detected recurrence (range)	Median survival time after primary surgical treatment (range)
Asymptomatic patients	8 months (3–24)	12 months (7–30)
Symptomatic patients	4 months (1–16)	14 months (5–34)

Surgical University Clinic, Heidelberg.

Table 5A. Type of surgical treatment for recurrence of gastric carcinoma

		No resection		
	Resection	Bypass anastomosis	Exploratory laparotomy	Other
Papachristou and Fortner, 1981[a]	19%	–	70%	29%
Suzuki et al, 1983[b]	27%	55%	8%	10%
Meyer and Pichlmayr, 1984[c]	20%	49%	68%	8%
Wenzl et al, 1987[d]	10%	27%	–	63%

[a] Papachristou DN, Fortner JG: Local recurrence of gastric adenocarcinomas after gastrectomy. J Surg Oncol 1981;18:47.

[b] Suzuki H, Endo M, Nakayama K: A review of the five-year survival rate and clinicopathologic factors in stomach cancer treated by surgery alone. Intern Advances Surg Oncol 1983;6:271.

[c] Meyer H-J, Pichlmayr R: Möglichkeiten und Grenzen der chirurgischen Therapie beim Magenkarzinomrezidiv: Ergebnisse nach 120 Reinterventionen. Langenbecks Arch Chir 1984;445.

[d] Wenzl E, Feil W, Schiessel R: Wert einer konsequenten Nachsorge beim Magenkarzinom. Wien Klin Wschr 1987;12:420.

Table 5B. Surgical treatment for recurrence of gastric carcinoma

	Resection	Palliative surgery without resection	Exploratory laparotomy
Follow-up group, authors' clinic	–	3/33 (9%)	4/33 (12%)
Referred patients with recurrent tumor	5/17 (29%)	5/17 (29%)	4/17 (24%)

Surgical University Clinic, Heidelberg.

consequences or prognostic advantages. The opportunity for a second resection was never realized. In contrast, some earlier reports indicated as well that a second resection was possible in an average of 20% of patients with recurrent gastric cancer.[6,8,14,15]

How can these poorer results be explained? We believe they stem from the fact that the group of patients receiving follow-up care in this series comprised individuals who had undergone total gastrectomies as primary treatment of their gastric cancer. Repeated surgery following detection of a local tumor recurrence is virtually impossible following total gastrectomy, however.[8,12,16] In general, resections may be carried out only in the case of gastric wall or anastomosis recurrence following partial gastric resection.[1,11,15] We were also able to achieve the generally indicated resection rates in patients referred to us for recurrent cancer of the gastric remnant (Tables 5A and 5B). The therapeutic benefit derived thereof should not be overestimated, however.[1,10,14,15] This holds true for the detection of metastases in asymptomatic patients as well, since the therapeutic possibilities available today are apparently ineffective in this situation. Early detection of metastases in cases of gastric carcinoma is therefore extremely problematical, not least from a psychological standpoint.[8,16]

Particularly in gastric carcinoma patients who have undergone total gastrectomies we should refrain from narrow, rigid, and expensive follow-up care and essentially focus our attention on the detection and treatment of postoperative conditions. Independently of this, however, precise patient follow-up examinations will continue to constitute the most important basis for quality control as well as for the assessment of surgical techniques and additional therapeutic procedures.

References

1. Herfarth C, Schlag P, Hohenberger P: Therapeutische Möglichkeiten bei locoregionären Rezidiven der Carcinome des Gastrointestinaltraktes. Chirurgie 1985;56:492.
2. Meyer H-J, Pichlmayr R: Patterns of recurrence in relation to therapeutic strategy in gastric cancer. Scand J Gastroenterol 1987;2 (suppl 133):45.
3. Schlag P, Herfarth C: Beziehung zwischen Ausdehnung des operativen Primäreingriffs und Häufigkeit lokoregionärer Rezidive, in Rohde H, Troidl H (eds): Das

Magenkarzinom: Methodik klinischer Studien und therapeutischer Ansätze. Stuttgart, Georg Thieme, 1984, p. 138.
4. Huchzermeyer H, Meyer H-J: Die Nachsorge des magenresezierten Patienten, in Langhans P, Meyer H-J, Pichlmayr R (eds): Aktuelle Therapie des Magenkarzinoms. Berlin-Heidelberg-New York, Springer, 1985, p. 181.
5. Schlag P: Nachsorge des operierten Magenkarzinompatienten. Probleme beim magenlosen Patienten. Klinikarzt 1978;7:397.
6. Papachristou DN, Fortner JG: Local recurrence of gastric adenocarcinomas after gastrectomy. J Surg Oncol 1981;18:47.
7. Koga S, Kishimoto H, Tanaka K, et al: Clinical and pathologic evaluation of patients with recurrence of gastric cancer more than five years postoperatively. Am J Surg 1978;136:317.
8. Metzger U, Küpfer A, Hollinger A, et al: Tumornachsorge beim radikal operierten Magenkarzinom. Eine prospektive Studie, in Häring R (ed): Therapie des Magenkarzinoms, Ed Medizin. Basel, Weinheim, 1984, p. 433.
9. Quentmeier A, Schlag P, Schmidt-Gayk H, et al: Ca 19-9 und CEA: Fortschritt bei der Diagnose und Verlaufsbeobachtung des Magencarcinoms durch kombinierte Bestimmung zweier Tumormarker. Langenbecks Arch Chir 1984;(Congress report):540.
10. Schlag P, Buhl K, Beck J, et al: Indikationen und Möglichkeiten operativer Therapie beim Magenkarzinomrezidiv, in Langhans P, Meyer H-J, Pichlmayr R (eds): Aktuelle Therapie des Magenkarzinoms. Berlin-Heidelberg-New York, Springer, 1985, p. 129.
11. Allum WH, Hockey MS, Fielding JW: Gastric remnant recurrence – detection and implications for the management of gastric cancer. Clin Oncol 1984;10:333.
12. Schwemmle K, Helling HJ: Onkologische Nachsorge und chirurgische Therapie von Lokalrezidiv und Metastasen beim Magencarcinom, in Gall FP, Hermanek P, Hornig D (eds): Magenkarzinom: Epidermiologie, Pathologie, Therapie, Nachsorge. Munich, W Zuckschwerdt, 1986, p. 189.
13. Viste A, Rygh AB, Soreide O: Cancer of the stomach – is a follow-up program of any importance for the patient? Clin Oncol 1984;10:325.
14. Wenzl E, Feil W, Schiessel R: Wert einer konsequenten Nachsorge beim Magenkarzinom. Wien Klin Wschr 1987;12:420.
15. Suzuki H, Endo M, Nakayama K: A review of the five-year survival rate and clinicopathologic factors in stomach cancer treated by surgery alone. Intern Advances Surg Oncol 1983;6:271.
16. Schlag P, Merkle P, Herfarth C: Neue Aspekte in der Konzeption adjuvanter und nachsorgender Therapie des Magencarcinoms? Chirurg 1979;50:432.

Part IV
Chemotherapy of Gastric Carcinoma

CHAPTER 10

Polychemotherapy of Gastric Carcinoma

H. Wilke, P. Preusser, W. Achterrath, H.-J. Schmoll, U. Fink, and H. Poliwoda

Introduction

Gastric carcinoma is the second leading cause of death due to malignant neoplasias in the Federal Republic of Germany; 28 deaths per 100,000 inhabitants are recorded every year.[1]

The following 5-year survival rates in terms of AJCC stages[2] were achieved through surgical treatment alone: stage I, 65%; stage II, 22%; stage III, 5%; and stage IV, 0%.[3]

The survival rate for patients who have liver metastases and who do not undergo surgical and cytostatic treatment averages 4 to 6 months, and, in cases of peritoneal carcinosis, 4 to 6 weeks.[4–6] Patients with measurable tumor parameters survive an average of 4 months following a palliative operation and 6 months after clinically complete tumor resection.[7,8]

Gastric carcinoma is already disseminated in approximately 75% of all patients at diagnosis.[9–14] Only unsatisfactory results are therefore achieved by means of regional treatment procedures (surgery and/or radiation therapy). Of all therapeutic measures, preference should therefore be given to a systemic treatment (cytostatic agents).

Only few cytostatic agents induce response rates of >15% in patients with advanced gastric cancer without prior chemotherapy (Table 1). In chemotherapy of refractory gastric carcinoma ADM,[15,16] TZT,[17] and CDDP[18–24] resulted in remission rates ranging from 15% to 20%.

Polychemotherapy

Numerous combinations of cytostatic agents were tested in advanced cases of gastric carcinoma, with two to four substances of proven effectiveness being combined most of the time. The following factors complicate any retrospective comparison between published studies:

Table 1. Single agent activity in gastric carcinoma without previous chemotherapy (>15% remissions)

Drug	Patients (n)	CR n	CR %	CR + PR n	CR + PR %	Study
5-FU	54	1	2	11	20	a,b,c,d
ADM	124	10	8	21	17	d,e,f,g
Epi-ADM	39	2	5	8	21	h
CDDP	14	2	14	5	36	i
Etoposide	14	0		3	21	j
MTC	211	NA		63	30	k,l
BCNU	55	1	2	10	18	d,m

[a] Cocconi G, DeLisi V, Di Blasio B: Randomized comparison of 5-FU alone or combined with mitomycin and cytarabine (MFC) in the treatment of advanced gastric cancer. Cancer Treat Rep 1982;66:1263.
[b] DeLisi V, Cocconi G, Tonato M, et al: Randomized comparison of 5-FU alone or combined with carmustine, and mitomycin (BAFMi) in the treatment of advanced gastric cancer: a phase III trial of the Italian Clinical Research Oncology Group (GOIRC). Cancer Treat Rep 1986;70:481.
[c] Kolaric K, Potrebica V, Stanovnik M: Controlled phase III clinical study of 4-epi-doxorubicin + 5-fluorouracil versus 5-fluorouracil alone in metastatic gastric and rectosigmoid cancer. Oncology 1986;43:73.
[d] MacDonald JS, Gunderson LL, Cohn I Jr: Cancer of the stomach, in DeVita VT, Hellman S, Rosenberg SA (eds): Cancer, Principles and Practice of Oncology. Lippincott, Philadelphia, 1985, p 534.
[e] The Gastrointestinal Tumor Study Group: Phase II-III chemotherapy studies in advanced gastric cancer. Cancer Treat Rep 1979;63:1871.
[f] Levi JA, Fox RM, Tattersall MH, et al: Analysis of a prospective randomized comparison of doxorubicin versus 5-fluorouracil, doxorubicin, and BCNU in advanced gastric cancer: implications for future studies. J Clin Oncol 1986;4:1348.
[g] Moertel CG, Lavin PT: Phase II-III chemotherapy studies in advanced gastric cancer. Cancer Treat Rep 1979;63:1863.
[h] Walder S, Green M, Muggia F: The role of anthracyclines in the treatment of gastric cancer. Cancer Treat Rev 1985;12:105.
[i] Leichmann L, MacDonald B, Dindogru A, et al: Platinum: A clinical active drug in advanced adenocarcinoma of the stomach, abstract. Proc Amer Assoc Cancer Res 1982;110:430.
[j] Kelsen DP, Magill G, Cheng E, et al: Phase II trial of etoposide (VP16) in the treatment of upper gastrointestinal malignancies, abstract. Proc ASCO 1982;96:C-371.
[k] Comis RL: Mitomycin C in gastric cancer, in Carter SK, Crooke ST (eds): Mitomycin C – Current Status and New Developments. New York, Academic Press, 1979, p 129.
[l] Schein PS, MacDonald JS, Hoth D, et al: Mitomycin C: experience in the United States, with emphasis on gastric cancer. Cancer Chemother Pharmacol 1978;1:73.
[m] Moertel CG: Therapy of advanced gastrointestinal cancer with the nitrosoureas. Cancer Chemother Rep 1973;4:27.

- Varying dosage and application schedules, given in combinations of identical cytostatic agents
- Evaluation and definition of remission in previous studies without taking into account current standard criteria
- The admission of patients with varying prognostic factors.

Prognostic factors for which the response to chemotherapy is favorable include[25-28]:

Table 2. Combinations of two cytostatic agents

Combination	Patients (n)	CR n	CR %	CR + PR n	CR + PR %	mR (Mon)	mS (Mon)	Study
4-Epi-ADM/5-FU	32	1	3	13	41	8	NA	a
ADM/5-FU	95	0		4	18	NA	NA	b,c
ADM/MTC	76	5	7	17	22	5	4–5	d,e
5-FU/MTC	103	NA		25	24	3–3,5	4	f,g
5-FU/MeCCNU	180	NA		36	20	3	3	e,f
5-FU/BCNU	62	NA		19	31	10	7,7	f

[a] Kolaric K, Potrebica V, Stanovnik M: Controlled phase III clinical study of 4-epi-doxorubicin + 5-fluorouracil versus 5-fluorouracil alone in metastatic gastric and rectosigmoid cancer. Oncology 1986;43:73.

[b] Cullinan SA, Moertel CG, Fleming TR, et al: A comparison of three chemotherapeutic regimens in the treatment of advanced pancreatic and gastric carcinoma. JAMA 1985;12:2061.

[c] The Gastrointestinal Tumor Study Group: Randomized study of combination chemotherapy in unresectable gastric cancer. Cancer 1984;53:13.

[d] Dalley D, Erlichman C, Fine S: Treatment of advanced gastric carcinoma with mitomycin and doxorubicin. Cancer Treat Rep 1986;70:897.

[e] Douglass HO Jr, Lavin P, Goudsmit A, et al: An Eastern Cooperative Oncology Group evaluation of combinations of methyl-CCNU, mitomycin C, Adriamycin, and 5-fluorouracil in advanced measurable gastric cancer (EST 2277). J Clin Oncol 1984;2:1372.

[f] Earl HM, Coombs RC, Schein PS: Cytotoxic chemotherapy for cancer of the stomach. Clin Oncol 1984;3:351.

[g] O'Connell MJ: Current status of chemotherapy for advanced pancreatic and gastric cancer. J Clin Oncol 1985;3:1032.

- Good performance status
- Largely complete surgical reduction of primary tumor
- No distant metastases.

Unfavorable prognostic factors include[25,27,28]:

- Poor overall condition
- Nonresectable primary tumor
- Distant metastases (especially liver, lung, skeleton).

Combinations of Two Cytostatic Agents

5-FU was combined with anthracyclines, nitrosoureas, or mitomycin in more recent studies (Table 2). In five of six studies the results obtained with the combinations were no better than those achieved with the same cytostatic agents in single-drug therapy. The remission rates achieved with epidoxorubicin/5-FU were markedly higher than with ADM/5-FU in one study. This result is surprising, as epidoxorubicin and doxorubicin exhibit comparable activities in cases of gastric carcinoma.

Table 3. FAM protocol according to MacDonald[a]

5-FU	600 mg/g IV	Days 1, 8, 29, 36
ADM	30 mg/g IV	Days 1 and 29
MTC	10 mg/g IV	Day 1
Repeat every 8 weeks		

[a] MacDonald JS, Schein PS, Woolley PV, et al: 5-Fluorouracil, doxorubicin, and mitomycin (FAM) combination-chemotherapy for advanced gastric cancer. Ann Intern Med 1980;93:533. Reprinted with permission.

Combinations of Three Cytostatic Agents (FA-Based)

The development of the FAM protocol[29] (Table 3) was crucial in shaping polychemotherapy for gastric carcinoma. Currently employed more frequently in the treatment of advanced gastric carcinoma, the original FAM protocol produced complete remission rates ranging from 0% to 11% and overall remission rates of 8% to 44% with median duration of 5 to 9 months. Median survival for all patients was 6 to 7 months (Table 4). Discounting one study with a conspicuously low remission rate, no statistically significant difference was found in overall remission rates between the various studies.

Table 4. FAM protocol according to MacDonald: Seven studies with >14 patients

No. of patients	CR n	CR %	CR + PR n	CR + PR %	mR (Mon)	mS (Mon)	Reference
62	0		26	42	9	5,5	a
45	1	2	20	44	7	7+	b
46	2	4	18	39	5	6	c
33	2	6	7	21	NA	6	d
27	3	11	6	22	NA	5,5	e
64	NA		19	30	5	6	f
25	0		2	8	NA	6	g

[a] MacDonald JS, Schein PS, Woolley PV, et al: 5-Fluorouracil, doxorubicin, and mitomycin (FAM) combination-chemotherapy for advanced gastric cancer. Ann Intern Med 1980;93:533.
[b] Beretta G, Fraschini P, Labianca R, et al: The value of FAM polychemotherapy in advanced gastric carcinoma, abstract. Proc ASCO 1982;103:C-400.
[c] Douglass HO Jr, Lavin P, Goudsmit A, et al: An Eastern Cooperative Oncology Group evaluation of combinations of methyl-CCNU, mitomycin C, adriamycin, and 5-fluorouracil in advanced measurable gastric cancer (EST 2277). J Clin Oncol 1984;2:1372.
[d] Haim N, Cohen Y, Honigman J, et al: Treatment of advanced gastric carcinoma with 5-fluorouracil, adriamycin, and mitomycin C (FAM). Cancer Chemother Pharmacol 1982;8:277.
[e] Haas C, Oishi N, McDonald B, et al: Southwest Oncology Group phase II-III gastric cancer study: 5-fluorouracil, adriamycin, and mitomycin C + vincristine (FAM vs V-FAM) compared to chlorozotocin (CZT), M-AMSA, and dihydroxyanthracenedione (DHAD) with unimpressive differences, abstract C-478. Proc ASCO 1983;2:122.
[f] Pannettiere FJ, Haas C, McDonald B, et al: Drug combinations in the treatment of gastric adenocarcinoma: a randomized Southwest Oncology Group study. J Clin Oncol 1984;2:420.
[g] Biran H, Sulkes A: A possible dose-response relationship in FAM chemotherapy for advanced gastric cancer, abstract. Proc ASCO 1984;132:C-515.

Table 5. Intensified FAM: FAM2, interval reduction

Dosage	Patients (n)	CR n %	CR + PR n	CR + PR %	mR (Mon)	mS (Mon)	Study
5-FU 600 mg/g Days 1, 8, 22, 29	22	0	4	18	NA	6.8	a
ADM 30 mg/g Days 1 and 22							
MTC 10 mg/g Day 1 (every 6 weeks)							
5-FU 400 mg/g Days 1–3, 21–23	100	NA	35	35	9.5	9	b,c
ADM 40 mg/g Days 2 and 22							
MTC 10 mg/g Day 1 (every 6 weeks)							

[a] Haim N, Epelbaum R, Cohen Y, et al: Further studies in the treatment of advanced gastric cancer by 5-fluorouracil, adriamycin (doxorubicin), and mitomycin C (modified FAM). Cancer 1984;54:1999.

[b] Cartei G: 5-Fluorouracil, Adriamycin und Mitomycin C beim metastasierenden Magenkarzinom, in Nagel GA, Bach F, Bartsch HH (eds): Aktuelle Onkologie. Munich-Bern-Vienna, W. Zuckerschwerdt, 1985, p 56.

[c] Fornasiero A, Cartei G, Daniele O, et al: FAM2 regimen in disseminated gastric cancer. Tumori 1984;70:77.

Intensified FAM (FAM2)

During the intensified FAM protocols an attempt was made to increase the dosage of individual agents for each course of treatment indirectly by shortening the intervals. The goal was to increase the effectiveness of FAM (Table 5). In two studies with different dosage and application schedules, no improvement in the treatment result was found when a comparison was made to the original regimen (χ^2 test, $P > .05$).

FAM Variants

Various modifications of FAM were tested in six other studies, with a remission rate of 26%, median duration of remission of 5 to 9 months, and median survival time of 6 to 9 months (Table 6).

No statistically significant differences were found when treatment results (remission rates, median duration of remission, median survival time) achieved with the original FAM regimen and its modifications were compared. The same held true when 4-epidoxorubicin was substituted for ADM in the FAM protocol.[30]

Table 6. FAM modifications (studies with >14 patients)

Dosage	Patients (n)	CR n	CR %	CR + PR n	CR + PR %	mR (Mon)	mS (Mon)	Study
5-FU 600 mg/g Days 29–32 ADM 50 mg/g Day 3 MTC 10 mg/g (Every 8 weeks, sequentially)	63	NA		15	23	5	5.5	a
5-FU 275 mg/g Days 1-5, every 5 weeks ADM 30 mg/g Day 1, every 5 weeks MTC 10 mg/g Day 1, every 10 weeks	15	0		7	47	7	NA	b
Identical	18	0		3	17	NA	6.4	c
5-FU 350 mg/g ADM 20 mg/g MTC 8 mg/g Day 1, every 3 weeks	31	0		8	26	5.5+	NA	d
5-FU 600 mg/g Days 1–8, every 4 weeks ADM 30 mg/g Day 1, every 4 weeks MTC 10 mg/g (Every 8 weeks)	17	NA		4	24	9+	9+	e
5-FU 300 mg/g Days 1–5, 29–33 ADM 30 mg/g Days 1, 29 MTC 10 mg/g Day 1 (Every 8 weeks)	44	2	5	11	25	5.5	NA	f

[a] Pannettiere FJ, Haas C, McDonald B, et al: Drug combinations in the treatment of gastric adenocarcinoma: a randomized Southwest Oncology Group Study. J Clin Oncol 1984;2:420.

[b] The Gastrointestinal Tumor Study Group: Phase II-III chemotherapy studies in advanced gastric cancer. Cancer Treat Rep 1979;63:1871.

[c] The Gastrointestinal Tumor Study Group: Randomized study of combination chemotherapy in unresectable gastric cancer. Cancer 1984;53:13.

[d] Oshima K, Yamada T, Nonaka T, et al: Treatment of advanced GI cancer patients with 5-FU, Adriamycin, and mitomycin C (FAM), abstract 3977. Proc 13th Intern Cancer Congress, Seattle, 8–15 September 1982, p 665.

[e] Beretta G, Fraschini P, Labianca R, et al: Weekly 5-fluorouracil (F) versus combination chemotherapy for advanced gastrointestinal carcinoma. A perspective study program, abstract. Proc ASCO 1986;94:C-367.

[f] Kim NK: Chemotherapy of advanced gastric carcinoma with 5-fluorouracil, Adriamycin, mitomycin (FAM), and 5-fluorouracil, adriamycin, cisplatin (FAP) combinations: experience in Korea, in Ogawa M, Muggia FM, Rozencweig M (eds): Adriamycin, Its Expanding Role in Cancer Treatment. Amsterdam, Excerpta Medica, 1984, p 137.

Table 7. FAMe treatment results

Combination	Patients (n)	Studies (n)	CR n	CR %	CR + PR n	CR + PR %	mR (Mon)	mS (Mon)	Reference
FAMe	55	2	6	11	15	27	5	6	a,b

[a] Douglass HO Jr, Lavin P, Goudsmit A, et al: An Eastern Cooperative Oncology Group evaluation of combinations of methyl-CCNU, mitomycin C, adriamycin, and 5-fluorouracil in advanced measurable gastric cancer (EST 2277). J Clin Oncol 1984;2:1372.
[b] The Gastrointestinal Tumor Study Group: Phase II-III chemotherapy studies in advanced gastric cancer. Cancer Treat Rep 1979;63:1871.

FA Plus One Additional Cytostatic Agent

Several studies used combinations of ADM, nitrosoureas, CDDP, and MTX instead of FAM. The combinations FAMe, FAB, FAP, and FAMTX were tested on a larger group of patients.

FAMe (Table 7)

A remission rate of 27%, including 11% complete remissions, was achieved in 55 patients with the FAMe combination. The median remission duration lasted for 5 months, the median survival time was 6 months. In this study, the proportion of patients with favorable prognostic factors was relatively large. The primary tumor was resected prior to chemotherapy in 40% of the patients. In addition, a palpable decrease in the size of the liver was interpreted as remission.

FAB (Table 8)

FAB was employed in two prospective randomized studies and in two open clinical phase II studies. An overall remission rate of 43%, with a median duration of remission of 7 to 9 months and a median survival time of 6 to 8 months, were achieved in 177 patients. No statistically significant differences in the therapeutic results were found between the open and randomized studies.

FAP (Table 9)

FAP was tested in eight studies in different dosage and application schedules. A 36% remission rate, with a median remission duration of 5 to 7 months and a median survival time of 6 to 13 months, was attained.

Table 8. FAB studies with > 14 patients (4 studies)

No. of patients	CR n	CR %	CR + PR n	CR + PR %	mR (Mon)	mS (Mon)	Reference
17	0		4	24	NA	5.5	a
35	2	6	18	51	NA	NA	b
75	5	7	30	40	7	8	c
50	3	6	24	48	9	7	d,e

[a] Schnitzler G, Queisser W, Heim ME, et al: Phase III study of 5-FU and carmustine versus 5-FU, carmustine, and doxorubicin in advanced gastric cancer. Cancer Treat Rep 1986;70:477.
[b] Levi JA, Dalley DN, Aroney RS: Improved combination chemotherapy in advanced gastric cancer. Br Med J 1979;2:1471.
[c] Levi JA, Fox RM, Tattersall MH, et al: Analysis of a prospective randomized comparison of doxorubicin versus 5-fluorouracil, doxorubicin, and BCNU in advanced gastric cancer: implications for future studies. J Clin Oncol 1986;4:1348.
[d] Lopez M, DiLauro L, Papaldo P, et al: Treatment of advanced measurable gastric carcinoma with 5-fluorouracil, adriamycin, and BCNU. Oncology 1986;43:288.
[e] Lopez M, Perno CF, DiLauro L, et al: 5-Fluorouracil, adriamycin, BCNU (FAB) combination chemotherapy for advanced gastric cancer. Cancer Chemother Pharmacol 1984;12:194.

FAMTX (Tables 10 and 11)

5-FU, ADM, and MTX were tested in an identical dosage (5-FU 1.5 g/m²/day 1, ADM 30 mg/m²/day 14, MTX 1.5 g/m²/day 1, repeat after 4 weeks) in three clinical phase II studies and in two pilot studies (Table 10). The full remission rate was 11%, and overall remission rate was 43%. The median survival time in the phase II study was approximately 7 months.

In two other studies (Table 11), this combination was tested using dosages that differed from the original protocol (reduced dosage of 5-FU and MTX one time; lower MTX and higher 5-FU dosage the other). Differing results were obtained in these studies, with overall remission rates of 10% and 50%.

The original FAMTX protocol is currently being tested against FAM in a prospective randomized EORTC study. How FAMTX ranks among the other protocols will become known conclusively only at the end of this study.

Quadruple Combinations: FA + Two Additional Cytostatic Agents (Table 12)

Expanding the FAM protocol by BCNU, MeCCNU, chlorozotocin, or TZT did not lead to any improvement in therapeutic results in comparison to the original regimen.

Table 9. FAP studies with >14 patients (8 studies)

No. of patients	CR n	CR %	CR + PR n	CR + PR %	mR (Mon)	mS (Mon)	Reference
18	0		9	50	6+	12	a
16	1	6	6	38	NA	NA	b
17	3	18	9	53	NA	10	c
18	1	6	9	50	4.5	NA	d
26	3	12	13	50	7	9	e,f
35	0		10	29	5.5	6	g
41	1	17	7	17	6	NA	h
16	0		5	31	NA	13	i

[a] Wagener DJT, Yap SH, Wobbes T, et al: Phase II trial of 5-fluorouracil, adriamycin, and cisplatin (FAP) in advanced gastric cancer. Cancer Chemother Pharmacol 1985;15:86.

[b] Rougier P, Droz JP, Amiel JL, et al: Gastric carcinoma: a phase II trial of chemotherapy with association 5-fluorouracil (5 FU), adriamycin (ADR) and cisplatin (DDP) (FAP Protocol) in metastasized or inoperable patients. Preliminary results. Cancer Chemother Pharmacol 1985;14 (suppl):54.

[c] Woolley P, Smith F, Esteves R, et al: A phase II trial of 5-FU, adriamycin and cisplatin (FAP) in advanced gastric cancer, abstract. Proc ASCO 1981;455:C-481.

[d] Figoli F, Galligioni E, Crivellari D, et al: Cisplatin (DDP) in combination with adriamycin (A) and fluorouracil (F) (DAF) in advanced gastric cancer–a phase II study, abstract. Proc ASCO 1986;95:C-369.

[e] Moertel CG, Fleming T, O'Connell M, et al: A phase II trial of combined intensive course 5-FU, adriamycin and cis-platinum in advanced gastric and pancreatic carcinoma, abstract. Proc ASCO 1984;137:C-535.

[f] Moertel CG, Rubin J, O'Connell MJ, et al: A phase II study of combined 5-fluorouracil, doxorubicin, and cisplatin in the treatment of advanced upper gastrointestinal adenocarcinomas. J Clin Oncol 1986;4:1053.

[g] Cazap EL, Gisselbrecht C, Smith FP, et al: Phase II trials of 5-FU, doxorubicin, and cisplatin in advanced, measurable adenocarcinoma of the lung and stomach. Cancer Treat Rep 1986;70:781.

[h] Kim NK: Chemotherapy of advanced gastric cancer with 5-fluorouracil, Adriamycin, mitomycin (FAM), and 5-fluorouracil, adriamycin, cisplatin (FAP) combinations: experience in Korea, in Ogawa M, Muggia FM, Rozencweig M (eds): Adriamycin: Its Expanding Role in Cancer Treatment. Amsterdam, Excerpta Medica, 1984, p 137.

[i] Robinson E, Haim N, Epelbaum R, et al: Phase II trials in the treatment of advanced gastric cancer. I. 5-Fluorouracil, adriamycin and mitomycin (FAM). II. Cisplatin, Adriamycin and 5-fluorouracil (DAF), abstract. Proc ASCO 1985;77:C-300.

Combinations of Cytostatic Agents (Not FA-Based)

Cisplatin-Containing Combinations

The combinations CDDP/5-FU/BCNU and CDDP/5-FU/BCNU/mitomycin were tested by Kim and associates.[31,32] A remission rate of approximately 65% was achieved in both studies; however, the incomplete definition of remission and the excessively high percentage of patients who were not evaluable to statistical analysis detract from their informative value.

Table 10. FAMTX: Studies with >14 patients

No. of patients	CR n	CR %	CR + PR n	CR + PR %	mR (Mon)	mS (Mon)	Reference
100	12	12	59	59	NA	8	a
67	9	13	22	33	9	6	b
20	0		0		–	3.3	c

[a] Klein HO, Wickramanyake PD, Farrkh GR: 5-Fluorouracil (5-FU), adriamycin (ADM), and methotrexate (MTX)–a combination protocol (FAMTX) for treatment of metastasized stomach cancer, abstract. Proc ASCO 1986;84:C-325.

[b] Wils J, Bleiberg H, Dalesio O, et al: An EORTC gastrointestinal group evaluation of the combination of sequential methotrexate and 5-fluorouracil, combined with adriamycin in advanced measurable gastric cancer. J Clin Oncol 1987;4:1799.

[c] Herrmann R, Fritze D, Queisser W, et al: Chemotherapie des Magenkarzinoms. Dtsch med Wschr 1984;109:1704.

EAP (Tables 13 and 14)

EAP was tested in a disease-oriented phase II study in 56 patients with measurable tumors. The complete remission rate was 21%, and the overall remission rate was 73%.

A clinical complete remission could be confirmed pathohistologically in seven of 12 patients by "second-look" operations. The median duration of remission measured 7 months, whereas the median survival time for all patients was 9 months. The median survival time has not yet been reached after 26 months in patients with a clinically complete remission and in those with NED following surgical resection.

A comparison between the therapeutic results obtained with FAP and EAP shows that exchanging 5-FU for etoposide in the CDDP/ADM combination and/or changing the application schedule for ADM and CDDP results in a statistically significant increase in complete and overall remission rates (χ^2 test: $P<.01$ and .05, respectively). This is remarkable given the fact that only

Table 11. FAMTX: Variations with >14 patients

No. of patients	CR n	CR %	CR + PR n	CR + PR %	mR (Mon)	mS (Mon)	Reference
20	NA		10	50	5	NA	a
31	1	3	3	10	NA	5	b

[a] Scherdin G, Garbrecht M, Mullerleile U, et al: Polychemotherapy with methotrexate in medium dosage range, 5-fluorouracil and adriamycin in advanced gastric carcinoma. J Cancer Res Clin Oncol 1986;111(suppl):58.

[b] Muro H, Romero Acuna L, Castagnari A, et al: Sequential methotrexate, 5-fluorouracil (high dose) and doxorubicin for advanced gastric cancer. Cancer Treat Rep 1986;70:1333.

Table 12. FA + two additional cytostatic agents

Regimen	No. of patients	CR + PR (%)	mR (Mon)	mS (Mon)	Reference
FAMB	16	30	4	NA	a
BAFMi	41	22	10	10	b
BAFMi	18	50	NA	NA	c
Total	75	26			
FAMMe	35	24	NA	NA	d
FAMC	23	26	NA	NA	e
FAMT	18	22	NA	NA	f

[a] Beretta G, Fraschini P, Ravaioli A, et al: FAM/FAMB polychemotherapy for advanced carcinoma of the stomach (ACS): a randomized study. Proc ASCO 1983;2:C-514.
[b] DeLisi V, Cocconi G, Tonato M, et al: Randomized comparison of 5-FU alone or combined with carmustine, and mitomycin (BAFMi) in the treatment of advanced gastric cancer: A phase III trial of the Italian Clinical Research Oncology Group (GOIRC). Cancer Treat Rep 1986;70:481.
[c] Bernath AM, Thomsvard CT: Treatment of advanced gastric carcinoma with BCNU, adriamycin, 5-FU and mitomycin-C (BAFMi). Proc ASCO 1979;20:C-87.
[d] Karlin DA, Stroehlein JR, Bennets RW, et al: Phase I-II study of the combination of 5-FU, doxorubicin, mitomycin, and semustine (FAMMe) in the treatment of adenocarcinomas of the stomach, gastroesophageal junction, and pancreas. Cancer Treat Rep 1982;66:1613.
[e] Gisselbrecht C, Smith FP, MacDonald JS, et al: The effect of sequential addition of the nitrosourea, chlorozotocin to the FAM combination in advanced gastric cancer. Cancer 1983;51:1792.
[f] Ahlgren JD, Schmith FP, Harvey J, et al: A phase II study of FAM (5-FU, adriamycin and mitomycin-C) plus triazinate (T) for advanced measurable gastric cancer. Proc ASCO 1984;3:145.

Table 13. EAP protocol

ADM	20 mg/g IV	Days 1 and 7
CDPP	40 mg/g IV	Days 2 and 8
Etoposide	120 mg/g IV	Days 4, 5, 6

Dosage of etoposide reduced to 100 mg/g in patients aged ≥60 years

Repeat days 22–28

Table 14. EAP treatment results

No. of patients	CR (%)	CR + PR (%)	mR (Mon)	mS (Mon)	Reference
56	21	73	7	9	a

[a] Preusser P, Wilke H, Achterrath W, et al: Advanced gastric carcinoma: a phase II study with etoposide (E), adriamycin (A) and split course cisplatin (P) = EAP. Proc ASCO 1987;6:75.

Table 15. High-dose LV/5-FU: Some patients pretreated

Study	No. of patients	CR + PR (%)	mR (Mon)	mS (Mon)	Reference
1	27	48	NA	5.5	a
2	25	12	NA	6	b

[a] Machover D, Goldschmidt E, Chollet P, et al: Treatment of advanced colorectal and gastric adenocarcinomas with 5-fluorouracil and high-dose folinic acid. J Clin Oncol 1986;4:685.
[b] Arbuck SG, Douglass HO, Rrave F, et al: A phase II trial of 5-fluorouracil and high-dose intravenous leucovorin in gastric carcinoma. J Clin Oncol 1987;5:1150.

patients with one or more unfavorable prognostic factors (inoperable tumor and/or distant metastases) were admitted into the EAP study.

Currently, EAP is being subjected to a randomized trial versus FAM in patients with metastasized gastric carcinoma in a large multicentric study.

High-Dose Combinations Containing High-Dose Leucovorin/5-FU (Tables 15 and 16)

The high-dose LV/5-FU combination was tested in two studies which are difficult to compare because of considerable differences in dosages and application schedules.

The LV/5-FU/etoposide combination was developed for the treatment of patients older than 65 years and patients with heart disease.

In an ongoing phase II study this combination achieved a remission rate, average duration of remission, and survival time that were at least comparable to those obtained with FAM.

Prospective Randomized Studies (Tables 17 and 18)

Numerous combinations of cytostatic agents were tested against single drug therapy with 5-FU or ADM as the control in randomized studies (Table 17). In seven

Table 16. High-dose LV/5-FU/etoposide treatment results

No. of patients	CR (%)	CR + PR (%)	mR (Mon)	mS (Mon)	Reference
21	14	41	8	9.5	a,b

[a] Pannettiere FJ, Haas C, McDonald B, et al: Drug combinations in the treatment of gastric adenocarcinoma: a randomized Southwest Oncology Group Study. J Clin Oncol 1984;2:420.
[b] Wilke H, Preusser P, Fink U, et al: Preoperative "neoadjuvant" chemotherapy with etoposide/adriamycin/cisplatin (EAP) in local advanced gastric cancer. Proc ECCO 1987;4:32.

Table 17. Results of prospective randomized studies with 5-FU and ADM vs polychemotherapy

Regimen	No. of patients	CR + PR (%)	mS (Mon)	Reference
5-FU	30	20	NA	a
5-FU/Epi-ADM	32	41	NA	
5-FU	28	29	7.4	b
BCNU	23	17	3.5	
5-FU/BCNU	34	41	7.7	
5-FU	10	20	4.5	c
5-FU/MeCCNU	29	21	4.5	
5-FU	11	18	7.5	d
5-FU/ADM	11	27	7.0	
5-FU/ADM/MTC	13	38	7.5	
5-FU	14	21	10.0	e
5-FU/ADM/MTC	17	24	9+	
5-FU	41	15	7.0	f
5-FU/ADM/MTC/BCNU	41	22	7.0	
ADM	37	22	4.0	g
5-FU/MTC	53	32	4.5	
5-FU/MeCCNU	49	24	4.0	
ADM	70	13	5.0	h
5-FU/ADM/BCNU	75	40	8.0	

[a] Kolaric K, Potrebica V, Stanovnik M: Controlled phase III clinical study of 4-epi-doxorubicin + 5-fluorouracil versus 5-fluorouracil alone in metastatic gastric and rectosigmoid cancer. Oncology 1986;43:73.

[b] Kovach JS, Moertel CG, Schutt AJ: A controlled trial of combined 1,3-bis-(2-chloro-ethyl)-1-nitrosourea and 5-fluorouracil therapy for advanced gastric and pancreatic cancer. Cancer 1974;33:563.

[c] Baker LH, Vaitkevicius VK, Gehan E: Randomized prospective trial comparing 5-fluorouracil (NSC-19893) to 5-fluorouracil and methyl-CCNU (NSC-95441) in advanced gastrointestinal cancer. Cancer Treat Rep 1976;60:733.

[d] Cullinan SA, Moertel CG, Fleming TR, et al: A comparison of three chemotherapeutic regimens in the treatment of advanced pancreatic and gastric carcinoma. JAMA 1985;12:2016.

[e] Beretta G, Fraschini P, Labianca R, et al: Weekly 5-fluorouracil (F) versus combination chemotherapy for advanced gastrointestinal carcinomas. A prospective study program, abstract. Proc ASCO 1986;94:C-367.

[f] DeLisi V, Cocconi G, Tonato M, et al: Randomized comparison of 5-FU alone or combined with carmustine, and mitomycin (BAFMi) in the treatment of advanced gastric cancer: A phase III trial of the Italian Clinical Research Oncology Group (GOIRC). Cancer Treat Rep 1986;70:481.

[g] Moertel CG, Lavin PT: Phase II-III chemotherapy studies in advanced gastric cancer. Cancer Treat Rep 1979;63:1863.

[h] Lagunova IG, Cybulskij BA, Minerva OD, et al: Aufeinander folgende Strahlentherapie mit einem 25-meV Betatron und Chemotherapie mit Fluorouracil zur Behandlung von Kranken mit fortgeschrittenem Krebs des oberen Magenabschnittes. Radiobiol Radiother 1978;13:307.

Table 18. FMC: 3 Studies

No. of patients	CR + PR (%)	mS (Mon)	References
71	20	5–10	a,b,c

[a] Aaoyama M, Hirose H, Adachi N, et al: Comparison of combination therapy of 5-fluorouracil, mitomycin C and adriamycin (FAM) and mitomycin C, 5-fluorouracil and cytosine arabinoside (MFC) for advanced gastric cancer. Gan To Kagaku Ryoko 1981;8:757.
[b] Cocconi G, DeLisi V, De Blasio B: Randomized comparison of 5-FU alone or combined with mitomycin and cytarabine (MFC) in the treatment of advanced gastric cancer. Cancer Treat Rep 1982;66:1263.
[c] O'Connell MJ, Moertel CG, Lavin PT: Adriamycin (A), 5-fluorouracil + mitomycin C–cytosine arabinoside (FMC), and 5-fluorouracil + adriamycin + methyl CCNU (FAMe) in advanced gastric carcinoma, abstract. Proc ASCO 1978;19:C-146.

of eight studies no statistically significant differences in the therapeutic results (remission rate, median survival time) were found in patients with measurable tumors. Only in one study was the remission rate statistically significantly higher and the median duration of remission and survival time significantly longer with the FAB combination than with the ADM.

The FMC combination was tested in three randomized studies (Table 18). Treatment results in the control group (FAM; FAMe) were more favorable in two studies. In one study, no differences with respect to single-drug therapy were found in response and survival rates between FMC and 5-FU. These results indicate that, at least in this combination, ARA-C appears to be ineffective.

Adjuvant Chemotherapy (Table 19)

Cytostatic agents and polychemotherapy programs were employed in the capacity of an adjuvant treatment in patients with gastric carcinoma who underwent curative resection.

In 10 of 11 studies (without the FAM combination) of more than 100 patients per study, working groups from Europe and the United States found no significant differences in survival times between individuals treated with chemotherapy and the untreated control group. The combination 5-FU/MeCCNU was tested against an untreated control group in five studies. Only the GITSG found a significantly higher percentage of survivors after 4 years in the chemotherapy group compared with the untreated control group. Patients derived no benefit from chemotherapy in any of the other studies.

Adjuvant treatment with FAM was tested against an untreated control group in three prospective randomized studies (Mid-Atlantic Oncology Group, SWOG, Schein). To date, the results from two of the studies have been published. No significant difference in survival time was discovered between patients treated with FAM and the control group in either study.[33,34] Numerous randomized studies varying in design and chemotherapy protocols were published by Japa-

Table 19. Adjuvant chemotherapy (without FAM study) vs surgical treatment

Treatment	No. of patients	Significance	Reference
TSPA/Control	194	NS	a
FUdR/Control	397	NS	b
5-FU + MeCCNU/Control	156	NS	c
5-FU + MeCCNU/Control	142	$P < .03$	d
MTC/TSPA/Control	209	NS	e
MTC/Cyclophosphamide + Chromomycin A3/Control	350	NS	e
MTC + 5-FU/Periop MTC + 5-FU/Control	460	NS	e
5-FU + MTC Placebo	411	NS	f
5-FU + MeCCNU Control	180	NS	g

[a] Dixon WJ, Longmire WP, Holden WD: Use of triethylenethiophosphoramide as an adjuvant to the surgical treatment of gastric and colorectal carcinoma: ten year follow-up. Ann Surg 1971;173:16.
[b] Serlin O, Wolkoff JS, Amadeo JH, et al: Use of 5-fluorodeoxyuridine (FUdR) as an adjuvant to the surgical management of carcinoma of the stomach. Cancer 1969;24:223.
[c] Higgins GA, Amadeo JH, Smith DE, et al: Efficacy of prolonged intermittent therapy with combined 5-FU and methyl-CCNU following resection for gastric carcinoma. Cancer 1983;52:1105.
[d] Gastrointestinal Tumor Study Group: Controlled trial of adjuvant chemotherapy following curative resection for gastric cancer. Cancer 1982;49:1116.
[e] Koyama Y, Kimura T: Controlled clinical trials of chemotherapy as an adjuvant to surgery in gastric carcinoma. Proc 2nd Int Cancer Congr Buenos Aires, 1978, p 1.
[f] Fielding JWL, Fagg SL, Jones BG, et al: An interim report of a prospective randomized controlled study of adjuvant chemotherapy in operable gastric cancer. World J Surg 1983;7:390.
[g] Engstrom P, Lavin PT, Douglass HO, et al: Postoperative adjuvant 5-fluorouracil plus methyl-CCNU therapy for gastric cancer patients. Cancer 1985;55:1868.

nese groups. Even in these studies, during the course of which 5-FU and MTC were often employed, patients did not derive any benefit from the adjuvant chemotherapy.[35,36]

Combined Treatment with Chemotherapy and Radiotherapy

Combination chemo- and radiotherapy was tested in open studies and in a prospective randomized study.[37–45] Retrospective comparisons among the open studies demonstrate higher remission rates[40] and median survival times[34,41,46] after treatment with 5-FU plus radiation therapy than radiation therapy alone.[34,40,41,46] Median survival time was 13 months for radiotherapy plus 5-FU and 6 months for radiotherapy alone.[34,41,46] Twelve percent of the patients who underwent combined treatment were still alive 5 years later, whereas none of the control patients treated with radiation alone survived.[34,41,46]

FAM was administered together with sequential irradiation in three open studies.[43,44,45] Only the results of one study with a heterogeneous patient population (inoperable primary tumor, residual tumor following surgery, completely resected tumor in high-risk patients) have been published to date.[45] The median survival time in this study was 13 months.

Simultaneous chemotherapy (5-FU) and radiotherapy followed by subsequent maintenance treatment (5-FU + MeCCNu) was tested against chemotherapy alone (5-FU + MeCCNU) in patients with inoperable or residual gastric carcinomas during a prospective randomized study conducted by the GITSG.[42] Sixteen percent of patients treated simultaneously with chemotherapy and radiotherapy were still alive 5 years later, whereas 7% of the patients receiving chemotherapy alone survived.

The effect that prognostic factors have on survival time was examined in this study within the framework of a multivariate analysis.[42] Patients who underwent a resection of the primary tumor lived for a significantly longer period of time than did patients with a nonresectable tumor. Other factors such as age, gender, overall condition, and weight loss prior to the initiation of therapy, histology, localization of the primary tumor, and extent of the residual disease were not prognostically important.

At the present point in the examinations, additional randomized studies are necessary to establish the advantage of combined chemotherapy and radiation therapy over chemotherapy alone.

Discussion

The prognosis for patients with gastric carcinomas is particularly unfavorable. Longer term disease-free survival can only be achieved in a small percentage (10%) of patients with regional treatment procedures. Palliative measures for most patients consist of surgery, radiotherapy, and chemotherapy.

Many therapists still view gastric carcinoma as being only moderately responsive to chemotherapy. This opinion is reflected in turn by the number of patients currently being treated with chemotherapy in clinical studies (approximately 5%).

The reasons for restraint in using chemotherapy in cases of gastric carcinoma are complex:

- More than half of all patients are over 65 years of age. Tumor-induced secondary diseases (cardiovascular, pulmonary, hepatic, renal, etc) are frequent in this age group. For this reason more intensive and hence possibly more effective chemotherapy protocols often cannot be employed.
- Advanced gastric carcinomas in many cases lead to a rapid deterioration in the overall condition and to intraabdominal complications, so that intensive cytostatic therapy cannot be carried out.
- Approximately 30% overall remissions, and, rarely, complete remissions are achieved with the more frequently employed "standard combinations" (FAM and its modifications). Only complete remissions normally provide an opportunity for longer term disease-free survival in advanced cases, especially in metastasized tumor stages.

- Only a slight increase in life expectancy (7 months) was generally achieved in treated compared with untreated patients (4 months).
- Only a handful of prognostic factors relating to chemotherapy in cases of gastric carcinoma have been well defined to date. Clinical and experimental knowledge about the biological behavior of gastric carcinomas (influence of histology, oncogenes, growth kinetics, resistance developments) is insufficient. The differential application of cytostatic agents is therefore possible only on a restricted basis at the present time.

Despite these historical data, the attitude toward chemotherapy of gastric carcinoma should not be one of resignation. Rather, emphasis should be placed on the promising results obtained with recent combinations of cytostatic agents (FAMTX, EAP) and combined therapeutic procedures. To this end a critical analysis of the most important results from chemotherapy and trials is necessary.

Open Studies

A comparison of treatment results achieved with the combinations of cytostatic agents (FAM and its modifications: FAB, FAP, FAMTX, EAP) on sufficient numbers of patients showed that within the 95% confidence limits, FAB, FAMTX, and EAP produced clearly higher overall remission rates than did FAM and FAP. With the exception of EAP, none of the combinations cited resulted in more than 15% complete remissions. This is of particular importance, since primarily patients with unfavorable prognostic factors (measurable tumor parameter, metastasized stages) were treated in the EAP study. The considerable differences in the remission rates observed given an identical therapy protocol (FAM, FAB, FAP, FAMTX) may in part be explained by the large number of patients with favorable prognostic factors in the individual studies. The fact that no significantly different increases in survival time were achieved in the individual studies despite the varying overall remission rates may in part be explained by the:

- Absence of uniform criteria for inclusion
- Varying criteria for the assessment of remission (especially prior to 1980)
- Lack of information about any second-line treatments which may have been carried out
- Rare induction of complete remissions. A significant increase in survival time is not to be expected for the overall group if almost exclusively partial remissions are induced.

Prospective Randomized Studies

Treatment results (remission rates, median remission duration, median survival time) achieved in patients with measurable tumor parameters were statistically better with the FAB combination than with single-drug therapy using ADM in only one of the prospective randomized studies[47] which tested single-drug therapy against polychemotherapy.

The following factors must be judged critically when analyzing these results, however:

- The number of patients per therapy group was too low to statistically support differences in the remission rates of 10% to 20%.[48,49]
- The number of patients per therapy group was too low to statistically support significant differences in the median remission duration and survival time.[48,49]
- Stratification by prognostic factors was rarely carried out.
- The dosages were often reduced in the more effective combinations of cytostatic agents in comparison to single-drug therapy.[50–52]

Adjuvant Chemotherapy

In only one study[53] with adjuvant chemotherapy did average survival time increase in comparison to the untreated control group. The primary cause for these negative results is probably related to the excessively low to insufficient antineoplastic activity of these cytostatic agents and their combinations.

Based on the aforementioned results, no justified indication for adjuvant chemotherapy outside of trials exists to date. The question as to whether the indication for adjuvant chemotherapy will be changed when newer, more effective, combinations of cytostatic agents become available can be answered only by future well-planned studies.

Conclusions and Consequences

More recent treatment results (FAMTX, EAP) indicate that gastric carcinoma can be classified as a chemotherapy-sensitive tumor. Despite the still primarily palliative nature of chemotherapy in cases of gastric carcinoma, tumor-induced symptoms (pains, passage disorders, loss of appetite) of the latter may be reduced considerably and life expectancy increased with this treatment. That effective chemotherapy protocols (EAP) alone and especially in combination with surgery[54] may be employed even curatively seems conceivable based on the pathologically induced complete remissions obtained. These heartening initial results should intensify the treatment of patients within the framework of prospective collaborative therapy studies with surgeons, pathologists, and internal oncologists. One such concept is currently being pursued by the Interdisciplinary Study Group for Gastrointestinal Tumors.

Treatment results obtained in cases of gastric carcinoma could be improved by the:

- Development of new effective cytostatic agents
- Optimization of dosage and application schedules for effective cytostatic agents in single-drug and combination therapy[55]

- Differential application of cytostatic agents based on tumor biology and clinical prognosis.

To achieve this requires intensified experimental research in the area of tumor biology, development of suitable predictive testing systems relating to the response to chemotherapy, intensified clinical studies, and testing of effective polychemotherapy protocols combined with surgery (adjuvant, neoadjuvant), with or without radiotherapy.

References

1. Causes of Death 1983, in Federal Office of Statistics, Wiesbaden: Gesundheitswesen, Series 12. Stuttgart, W. Kohlhammer, 1984, p. 12.
2. UICC: Spiesse B, Hermanek P, Scheibe O, et al (eds): TNM-Atlas. Berlin-Heidelberg-New York, Springer, 1985, p. 90.
3. Diehl JT, Herrmann RE, Cooperman AM, et al: Gastric carcinoma. A ten year review. Ann Surg 1983;198:9.
4. Bengmark S. Jeppson B: Staging of liver metastases, in Wess L, Gilberg HA (eds): Liver Metastases. Boston, GK Hall, 1982, p. 268.
5. Koyama Y, Sugimachi K. Soejima K: Evaluation of extensive lymph node dissection for carcinoma of the stomach. World J Surg 1981;5:241.
6. Nekajima T, Harashima S, Hirata M: Prognostic and therapeutic values of peritoneal cytology in gastric cancer. Acta Cytol 1978;22:225.
7. De Lisi V, Cocconi G, Tonato M, et al: Randomized comparison of 5-FU alone or combined with carmustine, and mitomycin (BAFMi) in the treatment of advanced gastric cancer: a phase III trial of the Italian Clinical Research Oncology Group (GOIRC). Cancer Treat Rep 1986;70:481.
8. O'Connell MJ: Current status of chemotherapy for advanced pancreatic and gastric cancer. J Clin Oncol 1985;3:1032.
9. Borchard F, Sons HU: Klassifizierung des Magenkarzinoms aus pathologisch-anatomischer Sicht. Therapiewoche 1985;35:161.
10. Clarke JS, Cruze K, El Farra S, et al: The natural history and results of surgical therapy for carcinoma of the stomach. An analysis of 250 cases. Am J Surg 1961;102:143.
11. Dupont JB, Lee JR, Burton GR, et al: Adenocarcinoma of the stomach: review of 1497 cases. Cancer 1978;41:941.
12. Walther H: Krebsmetastasen. Basel, Schwabe, 1948, p 363.
13. Warren S: Studies on tumor metastasis: IV. Metastases of cancer of the stomach. N Engl J Med 1933;209:825.
14. Warwick M: Analysis of one hundred and seventy-six cases of carcinoma of the stomach submitted to autopsy. Ann Surg 1928;88:216.
15. Moertel CG, Lavin PT: Phase II-III chemotherapy studies in advanced gastric cancer. Cancer Treat Rep 1979;63:1863.
16. The Gastrointestinal Tumor Study Group: Phase II-III chemotherapy studies in advanced gastric cancer. Cancer Treat Rep 1979;63:1871.
17. Bruckner HW, Lokich JJ, Stablein DM: Studies of Bakers antifol, methotrexate and Razoxane in advanced gastric cancer. A Gastrointestinal Tumor Study Group Report. Cancer Treat Rep 1982;66:1713.
18. Aabo K, Pedersen H, Rorth M: Cisplatin in the treatment of advanced gastric carcinomas: a phase II study. Cancer Treat Rep 1985;69:449.

19. Beer M, Cocconi G, Ceci G, et al: A phase II study of cisplatin in advanced gastric cancer. Eur J Cancer Clin Oncol 1983;19:717.
20. Kantarjian H, Ajani JA, Karlin DA: Cis-diaminodichloroplatinum (II) chemotherapy for advanced adenocarcinoma of the upper gastrointestinal tract. Oncology 1985;42:69.
21. Lacave AJ, Wils H, Bleiberg E, et al: Advanced and chemotherapy-resistant gastric cancer (GC): benefit of additional MeCCNU (Me) and evaluation of CDDP (P), abstract. EORTC Symposium on Gastrointestinal Tract Cancer, Heidelberg, May 29–30, 1986.
22. Lacave AJ, Wils J, Diaz-Rubio E, et al: Phase II study of cisplatin (DDP) in chemotherapy resistant carcinoma of the stomach. Cancer Chemother Pharmacol 1985;14(suppl):39.
23. Perry MC, Green MR, Mick R, et al: Cisplatin in patients with gastric cancer: a cancer and leukemia group B phase II study. Cancer Treat Rep 1986;70:415.
24. Preusser P, Achterrath W, Niederle N, et al: Cisplatin. Arzneimitteltherapie 1985;2:50.
25. Bedikian AY, Chen TT, Khankhanian N, et al: The natural history of gastric cancer and prognostic factors influencing survival. J Clin Oncol 1984;2:305.
26. Bleiberg H: Prognostic significance of pathological staging in gastrointestinal tumors. Eur J Cancer Clin Oncol 1985;21:655.
27. Bruckner HW, Stablein DM: Sites of treatment failure: Gastrointestinal Tumor Study Group analyses of gastric, pancreatic, colorectal trials. Cancer Treat Rep 1983;2:199.
28. Lavin PT, Bruckner HW, Plaxe SC: Studies in prognostic factors relating to chemotherapy for advanced gastric cancer. Cancer 1982;50:2016.
29. MacDonald JS, Schein PS, Woolley PV, et al: 5-Fluorouracil, doxorubicin, and mitomycin (FAM) combination-chemotherapy for advanced gastric cancer. Ann Intern Med 1980;93:533.
30. Queisser W, Flechtner H, Heim ME, et al: 5-Fluorouracil, 4-epidoxorubicin, and mitomycin C (FEM) for advanced gastric carcinoma, a phase II trial. J Cancer Res Clin Oncol 1986;111(suppl):85.
31. Kim RH, Huh K, Ahn Y, et al: BCNU, cisplatin and 5-fluorouracil polychemotherapy in advanced gastric cancer. Proc ASCO 1985;4:95.
32. Kim RH, Kim CS: Chemotherapy of advanced gastric cancer with mitomycin C, BCNU, cisplatin and 5-fluorouracil in combination. Proc ASCO 1986;5:78.
33. Schein PS, Coombes RC, Chilvers C: For the international adjuvant trial in gastric cancer. A controlled trial of FAM (5-FU, doxorubicin, and mitomycin C) chemotherapy as adjuvant treatment for resected gastric carcinoma: an interim report. Proc ASCO 1986;5:79.
34. Galiano R, McCracken JD, Chen T: Adjuvant chemotherapy with 5-fluorouracil, Adriamycin, and mitomycin (FAM) in gastric cancer. Proc ASACO 1983;2:114.
35. Imanaga H, Nakazato H: Results of surgery for gastric cancer and effect of adjuvant mitomycin-C on cancer recurrence. World J Surg 1977;1:213.
36. Koyama Y: The current status of chemotherapy for gastric cancer in Japan with special emphasis on mitomycin-C. Rec Res Cancer Res 1978;63:135.
37. Asakawa H, Otawa K, Watari J: High energy x-ray therapy for stomach carcinoma, second report: the evaluation of radiotherapy for the early and the inoperable stomach carcinoma. Nippon Acta Radiol 1971;31:505.
38. Asakawa H, Takeda T: High energy x-ray therapy of gastric carcinoma. J Jap Soc Cancer Ther 1973;8:362.

39. Childs DS, Moertel CG, Holbrook MA, et al: Treatment of unresectable adenocarcinoma of the stomach with a combination of 5-fluorouracil and radiation. Am J Roentgenol 1986;102:541.
40. Falkson G: Halogenated pyrimidines as radiopotentiators in the treatment of stomach cancer. Prog Biochem Pharmacol 1965;1:695.
41. Falkson G, Falkson HC: :Fluorouracil and radiotherapy in gastrointestinal cancer. Lancet 1969;2:1252.
42. Gastrointestinal Tumor Study Group: A combination chemotherapy and combined modality therapy for locally advanced gastric carcinoma. Cancer 1982;49:1771.
43. Gunderson LL, Hoskins B, Cohen AM, et al: Combined modality treatment of gastric cancer. Int J Radiat Oncol Biol Phys 1983;9:965.
44. Haas L, Vaitkevicius V, Bukowski R, et al: Southwest Oncology Group (SWOG) pilot study of radiotherapy (R) + 5-fluorouracil (F) + Adriamycin = mitomycin C (M) in patients with minimal residual gastric cancer, abstract. Proc ASCO 1980;342:C-439.
45. Schein PS, Smith FP, Dritschillo A, et al: Phase I-II trial of combined modality FAM plus split-course radiation (FAM-RT-FAM) for locally advanced gastric and pancreatic cancer: a Mid-Atlantic Oncology Program Study, abstract. Proc ASCO 1983;126:C-491.
46. Lagunova IG, Cybulskij BA, Minerva OD, et al: Aufeinander folgende Strahlentherapie mit einem 24-meV Betatron und Chemotherapie mit Fluorouracil zur Behandlung von Kranken mit fortgeschrittenem Krebs des oberen Magenabschnittes. Radiobiol Radiother 1978;13:307.
47. Levi JA, Fox RM, Tattersall MH, et al: Analysis of a prospective randomized comparison of doxorubicin versus 5-fluorouracil, doxorubicin, and BCNU in advanced gastric cancer: implications for future studies. J Clin Oncol 1986;4:1348.
48. Gelber RD, Zelen M: Planning and reporting of clinical trials, in Calabresi PC, Schein PC, Rosenberg S (eds): Medical Oncology. New York, Macmillan, 1985, p 406.
49. Design and conduct of clinical trials, in DeVita VT, Hellman S, Rosenberg SA (eds): Cancer: Principles & Practice of Oncology. Philadelphia, JB Lippincott, 1985, p 329.
50. Cullinan SA, Moertel CG, Fleming TR, et al: A comparison of three chemotherapeutic regimens in the treatment of advanced pancreatic and gastric carcinoma. JAMA 1985;12:2061.
51. Kolaric K, Potrebica V, Stanovnik M: Controlled phase III clinical study of 4-epidoxorubicin + 5-fluorouracil versus 5-fluorouracil alone in metastatic gastric and rectosigmoid cancer. Oncology 1986;43:73.
52. Kovach JS, Moertel CG, Schutt AJ: A controlled trial of combined 1,3-bis-(2-chloroethyl)-1-nitrosourea and 5-fluorouracil therapy for advanced gastric and pancreatic cancer. Cancer 1974;33:563.
53. Gastrointestinal Tumor Study Group: Controlled trial of adjuvant chemotherapy following curative resection for gastric cancer. Cancer 1982;49:1116.
54. Wilke H, Preusser P, Fink U, et al: Preoperative "neoadjuvant" chemotherapy with etoposide/Adriamycin/cisplatin (EAP) in local advanced gastric cancer. Proc ECCO 1987;4:32.
55. Behre W, Brömsen J, Harstrick A, et al: Antitumor activity of anthracyclines in human gastric cancer xenografts depending on time scheduling. Blut 1987;55:224.

CHAPTER 11

Advanced Gastric Cancer: Results of Chemotherapy Trials of the EORTC Gastrointestinal Group

J.A. Wils

Introduction

In the past many patients with advanced gastric cancer were treated with chemotherapy because of the high response rates to combinations that were reported by the end of the 1970s. More recent data from randomized trials, however, have led researchers to question the value of applying combination chemotherapy routinely in advanced disease. Results from phase II and III studies conducted by the EORTC Gastrointestinal Group will be discussed, with implications for current treatment and future studies. Extensive reviews of the literature have been published elsewhere.[1,2]

EORTC Trial 40791

5-Fluorouracil has been the principal single agent used in the treatment of advanced disease for more than 20 years, and its response rate in collected series appears to be around 20%. Other drugs with reported activity include Adriamycin, mitomycin C, and the nitrosoureas, methyl-CCNU (Me) and BCNU.[3] Using combinations of these drugs, response rates ranging between 36% and 55% were reported,[4–8] and by the end of the 1970s the combinations of 5-FU, ADM, and mitomycin C (FAM), or F, ADM, and a nitrosourea, were considered successful regimens. At that time, because only a few randomized trials had been conducted with small patient samples, the contribution of Me or M to FA, which seemed to be the common denominator of all active regimens, was not apparent. Therefore the EORTC GI Group initiated a study to investigate the contribution of Me in the activity of MeFA by comparing this regimen with FA. MeFA was selected for this trial because it appeared to be the best therapeutic arm, especially according to data from GITSG as of 1979.[6]

A total of 189 patients were randomized to receive MeFA or FA. Stratification was made for measurable or nonmeasurable disease. Lesions detected solely by ultrasound or CT scanning were not considered measurable. Sixteen patients were not eligible, which left 173 patients, 57 of whom had measurable disease.

The response rate was 18% (5 of 28) with MeFA and 10% (3 of 29) with FA; median survival times were 32 and 21 weeks, respectively, (P = .14; log-rank test). We concluded that neither regimen can be recommended for the treatment of advanced gastric carcinoma.[9]

EORTC Trial 40793

In this trial we tested cisplatin in pretreated patients. The dose of CDDP was 100 mg/m^2 every 3 weeks. Thirty-four patients with measurable disease were entered into this phase II trial. Criteria for measurability were the same as those in EORTC trial 40791. Thirty-one patients were evaluable for response. Three complete and three partial responses (19%) with a median duration of 4 months were recorded. We concluded that CDDP was active in advanced gastric carcinoma, as previously reported,[10,11] and that further first-line investigations appeared to be justified.[12]

EORTC Trial 40841

In 1982 Klein and associates, employing sequential high-dose MTX and 5-FU combined with ADM (FAMTX), reported a 63% response rate in patients with advanced gastric carcinoma.[13] An update of this study reported that 59 of 100 patients responded, 10 completely, and the median survival time was 9 months for all patients. Three deaths due to toxicity occurred.[14]

We have conducted a multicenter phase II trial evaluating this protocol. MTX was given in a dose of 1500 mg/m^2 IV, followed after 1 hour by 5-FU, 1500 mg/m^2 IV, on day 1; LV rescue was started after 24 hours, 15 mg/m^2, orally, every 6 hours for 48 hours, and ADM, 30 mg/m^2 IV, was administered on day 15. Alkalinization of the urine before administering MTX and monitoring of the plasma MTX level was mandatory. Cycles were repeated every 4 weeks. CT scanning and ultrasound were accepted for the evaluation of disease in this study.

Of 65 eligible patients, 13 (20%) partially and nine (14%) completely responded; responses in three of these nine were documented histologically. Excluding early deaths, the response rate was 44%. Four toxic deaths occurred, although three were associated with major protocol violations. The median survival of all patients was 6 months. We concluded that the FAMTX regimen is active in gastric carcinoma, but that the toxicity, with or without protocol violations, appears to be considerable.[15]

EORTC Trial 40855

In an attempt to reduce the potential toxicity of FAMTX, yet maintain activity, a phase II study was initiated to investigate sequential MTX/5-FU in lower doses

Table 1. Toxicity of FAM vs FAMTX in advanced gastric carcinoma

	FAM	FAMTX
Nausea/vomiting median WHO grade (range)	1 (0–3)	1 (0–3)
WHO grade 3	4%	8%
Mucositis median WHO grade (range)	0 (0–2)	1 (0–3)
WHO grade 3	0%	8%
Diarrhea median WHO grade (range)	0 (0–3)	0 (0–2)
WHO grade 3	4%	0%
Alopecia (WHO grade 3)	24%	28%
WBC median nadir (range)	4.3×10^9 (0.1–13.9)	4.3×10^9 (0.7–12.4)
WHO grade 4	4%	4%
Thrombocytes median nadir (range)	$>100 \times 10^9$ (29–352)	$>100 \times 10^9$ (96–384)
WHO grade 4	4%	0%

and with a different time interval. MTX was administered in a dose of 300 mg/m^2 followed by 5-FU, 900 mg/m^2, after 7 hours.

The results were negative, with four partial responses in 28 patients and two severe toxicities,[16] suggesting that a lower dose of MTX can reduce the activity of sequential MTX/5-FU, but not the potential toxicity of MTX. Other trials investigating MTX/5-FU in different schedules all have yielded low response rates. Doses of MTX in these trials have ranged between 100 and 600 mg/m^2, doses of 5-FU between 600 and 1200 mg/m^2, and time intervals between 30 minutes and 24 hours. Response rates ranged between 0% and 21%.[17–19]

EORTC Trial 40851

To assess more precisely the toxicity of FAMTX we decided to initiate a randomized phase II trial comparing the toxicity of this regimen *v* FAM. A total of 69 patients had been entered as of February 1, 1987, and 50 were fully evaluable for toxicity studies. The results are depicted in Table 1.

The median number of cycles was one in FAM (range 1/2–2) and three in FAMTX (range 1–6). One toxic death occurred in the FAM arm; treatment was discontinued in one patient in the FAMTX arm because of toxicity. These data show that the toxicity of FAMTX is acceptable and fully comparable with that of FAM. This trial has now been extended to a randomized phase III trial, with evaluations of response rates and survival times in both treatment arms. By September 1, 1987, 100 patients were randomized. Updated toxicity data in 85 evaluable patients are virtually the same as those shown in Table 1. To detect a possible survival gain of 6 to 9 months, 200 patients must be accrued. Results of this trial will not be available until the end of 1988.

Discussion

Since the initial report from Georgetown University (Washington, DC, USA) first published in 1977 and updated in 1980 in combination with patients treated in France,[20] the FAM chemotherapy protocol has been adopted as "standard treatment" in advanced gastric cancer all over the world. In the majority of reported phase II trials the median survival times of responders have been compared with those of nonresponders, a comparison that is of limited value and that has been criticized severely.[21] In some trials survival times of all patients have been stated as ranging between 5 and 11 months.

Results of randomized trials, however, have questioned the superiority of combination chemotherapy over 5-FU alone. Results of multicenter phase III trials invariably have been inferior to those of single institution phase II studies. Randomized trials in advanced gastric cancer have compared different multidrug regimens or a multidrug regimen versus a single drug constituent. In three consecutive studies performed by GITSG, MeFA was found to produce the best results (response rates 7/15, 3/10, 4/16) compared with ADM or FAM, although the gain in median survival was only a few weeks.[6,22,23] The Southwest Oncology Group (SWOG) has conducted two trials with FAM in one of the arms. Response rates ranged between 22% and 30%, and median survival times were less than 6 months.[24,25] The study conducted by the Eastern Cooperative Oncology Group (ECOG) produced a 39% response rate for FAM and concluded that FAM should be strongly advocated for adjuvant treatment.[26] In two large trials, however, combination chemotherapy did not yield superior results when compared with 5-FU alone. The North Central Cancer Treatment Group (NCCTG) compared FAM with 5-FU (response rates 5/13 *v* 2/11, with median survival times of 7 months),[27] and in an Italian study[28] the combination of FAM and BCNU (BAFMI) was compared with 5-FU (response rates 9/41 *v* 6/41, median survivals of 6 vs. 7 months). Although reported response rates for MeFA in the literature generally fall within the 33% upper confidence limit of the results of our trial 40791, our results are in agreement with those of more recent randomized studies in which lower response rates have been reported for combination chemotherapy, particularly when more rigid response criteria for palpable, nonradiologically measurable disease are applied.

A constant finding in all studies employing FAM, MeFA, or FAB has been the low rate of complete responses, which for the most part has been <5%. Chemotherapy protocols with such low complete response rates and overall response rates of around 30% (mostly excluding early deaths, deaths due to toxicity, protocol violations, and losses to follow-up) are not likely to influence overall survival or benefit patients treated in an adjuvant setting. Although a difference in response rates between FAM and 5-FU alone has not been persuasively negated—because of small samples of patients with measurable disease—the benefit of FAM over 5-FU alone appears marginal. It is apparent that the median survival of patients with advanced gastric cancer does not exceed 6 months, and that combination chemotherapy has no beneficial effect on survival when compared with 5-FU alone.

Cisplatin has activity in gastric cancer and therefore has been added to FA (FAP). In six studies the response rates have ranged between 29% and 59%, and the median survivals from 4 to 12 months.[29-34] In some of these studies a histologically documented complete response has been reported. Because a randomized trial comparing FAP with FA plus triazinate or MeFA demonstrated a significant difference in survivals between FAP and FAT vs. MeFA,[35] FAP might be considered for further testing in randomized trials. On the other hand, because we have demonstrated that FA is not sufficiently active, CDDP has also been investigated in combination with 5-FU alone; of 31 patients, 14 responded, and the survival time for all patients was 10+ months.[36]

Another second-generation combination regimen (EAP) comprises etoposide (E), Adriamycin, and cisplatin. A response rate of 73% in 56 patients has been reported, including some histologically documented complete responses.[37] This protocol should certainly be investigated further in a randomized study.

Finally, the FAMTX regimen which yielded the best results we obtained in the treatment of advanced gastric carcinoma is now being investigated further in a randomized study. It has been stated that new protocols should have at least a response rate of 35% and a median survival time of 7 months in phase II trials, before being submitted to phase III testing.[38] Second-generation protocols such as FAP, EAP, and FAMTX are currently being tested by different groups in randomized trials and, it is hoped, will result in some progress in the treatment of advanced gastric cancer. For the time being, apart from 5-FU alone, chemotherapy in advanced gastric cancer should not be administered on a routine basis outside clinical trials.

References

1. O'Connell MJ: Current status of chemotherapy for advanced pancreatic and gastric cancer. J Clin Oncol 1985;3:1032.
2. Wils J: Current status of chemotherapy for advanced gastric cancer. Anticancer Res 1987;7:755.
3. Macdonald JS, Gunderson LL, Cohn I: Cancer of the stomach, in De Vita V, Hellman S, Rosenberg SA (eds): Cancer, Principles and Practice of Oncology. Philadelphia, JB Lippincott, 1982, p 534.
4. Lacave AJ, Brugarolas A, Buesa JM, et al: Methyl-CCNU (Me), 5-fluorouracil (F), adriamycin (A) (MeFA) versus MeF in advanced gastric cancer, abstract. Proc ASCO 1979;20:310.
5. Macdonald JS, Woolley PV, Smythe T, et al: 5-Fluorouracil, adriamycin and mitomycin-C treatment of advanced gastric cancer. Cancer 1979;44:42.

6. The Gastrointestinal Tumor Study Group: Phase II-III chemotherapy studies in advanced gastric cancer. Cancer Treatm Rep 1979;63:1871.
7. Levi JA, Dalley DN, Aroney RS: Improved combination chemotherapy in advanced gastric cancer. Br Med J 1979;2:1471.
8. Bitran JD, Desser RK, Koloff MF, et al: Treatment of metastatic pancreatic and gastric adenocarcinoma with 5-fluorouracil, adriamycin and mitomycin C (FAM). Cancer Treatm Rep 1979;63:2049.
9. Lacave AJ, Wils J, Bleiberg H, et al: An EORTC Gastrointestinal Group phase III evaluation of combinations of methyl-CCNU, 5-fluorouracil and adriamycin in advanced gastric cancer. J Clin Oncol 1987;5:1387.
10. Lacave AJ, Izarzugaza J, Anton-Aparicio LM, et al: Phase II clinical trial of cis-dichlorodiamine platinum in gastric cancer. Am J Clin Oncol 1983;6:35.
11. Leichman L, McDonald B, Dindogru A, et al: Cisplatin: an active drug in the treatment of disseminated gastric cancer. Cancer 1984;53:18.
12. Lacave AJ, Wils J, Diaz-Rubio E, et al: Cis-platinum as second-line chemotherapy in advanced gastric carcinoma. A phase II study of the EORTC Gastrointestinal Tract Cancer Cooperative Group. Eur J Clin Oncol 1985;21:1321.
13. Klein HO, Dias Wickramanayake P, Dieterle F, et al: Chemotherapie-protokoll zur Behandlung des metastasierenden Magenkarzinoms. Methotrexat, Adriamycin und 5-Fluorouracil. Dtsch Med Wschr 1982;45:1708.
14. Klein HO, Dias Wickramanayake P, Farrokh G-H: 5-Fluorouracil (5-FU), adriamycin (ADM) and methotrexate (MTX) – a combination protocol (FAMTX) for treatment of metastasized stomach cancer, abstract. Proc ASCO 1986;5:84.
15. Wils J, Bleiberg H, Blijham G, et al: An EORTC gastrointestinal group evaluation of the combination of sequential methotrexate (MTX) and 5-fluorouracil (F), combined with adriamycin (A) (FAMTX) in advanced measurable gastric cancer. J Clin Oncol 1986;4:1799.
16. Blijham G, Herrmann R, Neijt JP, et al: Background for and progress of an ongoing EORTC phase II study, abstract. Proc EORTC Symp on Gastrointest Cancer Update on Comb Modal Ther, Heidelberg, 1986.
17. Bruckner HW, Stablein DM: Single arm trials of triazinate, cisplatin and methotrexate combinations in advanced gastric cancer, abstract. Proc ASCO 1984;3:144.
18. Muro H, Romera Acuna L, Castagnari A, et al: Sequential methotrexate, 5-fluorouracil (high dose), and doxorubicin for advanced gastric cancer. Cancer Treatm Rep 1986;70:1333.
19. Ajani J, Levin B, Goudeau P, et al: Adriamycin with sequential methotrexate and 5-fluorouracil (AMF) for advanced gastric cancer, abstract. Proc ASCO 1986;5:93.
20. Macdonald JS, Schein PS, Woolley PV, et al: 5-Fluorouracil, doxorubicin and mitomycin C (FAM) combination chemotherapy for advanced gastric cancer. Ann Intern Med 1980;93:533.
21. Anderson JR, Cain KC, Gelber RD: Analysis of survival by tumor response. J Clin Oncol 1983;1:710.
22. The Gastrointestinal Tumor Study Group: A comparative clinical assessment of combination chemotherapy in advanced gastric carcinoma. Cancer 1982;49:1362.
23. The Gastrointestinal Tumor Study Group: Randomized study of combination chemotherapy in unresectable gastric cancer. Cancer 1984;53:13.
24. Panettiere FJ, Haas C, McDonald B, et al: Drug combinations in the treatment of gastric adenocarcinoma: a randomized Southwest Oncology Group study. J Clin Oncol 1984;2:420.

25. Haas C, Oistri N, McDonald B, et al: Southwest Oncology Group phase II-III gastric cancer study: 5-Fluorouracil, adriamycin and mitomycin-C + vincristine (FAM vs V-FAM) compared to chlorozotocin (CZT), m-AMSA and dihydroxyanthracenedine (DHAD) with unimpressive differences, abstract. Proc ASCO 1983;2:122.
26. Douglass HO, Lavin PT, Goudsmit A, et al: An Eastern Cooperative Oncology Group evaluation of combinations of methyl-CCNU, mitomycin-C, adriamycin and 5-fluorouracil in advanced measurable gastric cancer (EST 2277). J Clin Oncol 1984;2:1372.
27. Cullinan SA, Moertel CG, Fleming TR, et al: A comparison of three chemotherapeutic regimens in the treatment of advanced pancreatic and gastric carcinoma. Fluorouracil vs fluorouracil and doxorubicin vs fluorouracil, doxorubicin and mitomycin. JAMA 1985;253:2061.
28. De Lisi V, Cocconi G, Tonato M, et al: Randomized comparison of 5-FU alone or combined with carmustine, doxorubicin and mitomycin (BAFMi) in the treatment of advanced gastric cancer. A phase III trial of the Italian Clinical Research Oncology Group (GOIRC). Cancer Treatm Rep 1986;70:481.
29. Woolley PV, Smith F, Estevez R, et al: A phase II trial of 5-FU, adriamycin and cisplatin (FAP) in advanced gastric cancer, abstract. Proc ASCO 1981;22:455.
30. Vogl SE, Engstrom PF: Cisplatin, doxorubicin and 5-FU in combination for advanced gastric cancer. Cancer Treatm Rep 1984;68:1273.
31. Wagener DJTh, Yap SH, Wobbes Th, et al: Phase II trial of 5-fluorouracil, adriamycin and cisplatin (FAP) in advanced gastric cancer. Cancer Chemother Pharmacol 1985;15:86.
32. Moertel CG, Rubin J, O'Connell MJ, et al: A phase II study of combined 5-fluorouracil, doxorubicin and cisplatin in the treatment of advanced upper gastrointestinal adenocarcinomas. J Clin Oncol 1986;4:1053.
33. Rougier Ph, Droz JP, Piot G, et al: Phase II trial of combined 5-FU-adriamycin-cisplatin (FAP) in gastric carcinoma, abstract. Cancer Chemother Pharmacol 1986; 18(suppl 1):62.
34. Tagliagambe A, Lombardi M, Troiana R, et al: FAP regimen in advanced gastric cancer, abstract. Cancer Chemother Pharmacol 1986;18(suppl 1):67.
35. Bruckner HW, Stablein DM: A randomized study of 5-fluorouracil (F) and doxorubicin (A) with semustine (Me), cisplatin (P), or triazinate (T) for treatment of advanced gastric cancer, abstract. Proc ASCO 1986;5:90.
36. Lacave AJ, Anton-Aparicio L, Gonzales-Baron M, et al: Cisplatin and 5-fluorouracil (5FU) 120-hr infusion for advanced gastric cancer (GC): A phase II multicenter study, abstract. Proc ASCO 1987;6:91.
37. Preusser P, Wilke H, Achterrath W, et al: Advanced gastric carcinoma: A phase II study with etoposide (E), adriamycin (A) and split course cisplatin (P) = EAP, abstract. Proc ASCO 1987;6:75.
38. Killen JY, Ellenberg SS, Friedman MA: Combination chemotherapy (CT) regimens in advanced gastric cancer (GC), abstract. Proc ASCO 1985;4:82.

CHAPTER 12

Adjuvant Treatment of Gastric Cancer

J.A. Wils

Introduction

The incidence of gastric cancer has declined over the last 50 years in the western world, especially in the United States. The decline has been very steep—from 30 in 100,000 to 8 in 100,000—and for the most part has occurred in older people and in the white population. Gastric cancer now ranks as the sixth most common cause of death from cancer. In Western Europe the incidence is still around 20 in 100,000, while a higher incidence is found in Japan, South America (especially Chile), Eastern Europe, Spain, and Portugal. The downward trend, however, has been generally uniform, and even in Japan the incidence appears to be declining.

The prognosis of gastric cancer depends on the extent of the disease at presentation and consequently on whether a "curative" resection can be performed. Long-term survival or cure is possible only in those patients who have undergone complete resection for localized cancer. Five-year survival rate for all patients with gastric cancer is <10%, and, for the relatively small group of patients with localized disease resected for cure, 5-year survival rate is approximately 30%.

Lymph node status is an important prognostic sign. For patients without lymph node involvement 5-year survival is 40% to 60%, while for those with positive nodes no further than 3 cm from the primary (N1) 5-year survival is only 20% to 30%. Patients with tumors confined to the mucosa or submucosa (T1) without node invasion (stage I) carry the best prognosis, with a 5-year survival rate of approximately 80%, but patients with this early stage of gastric cancer are diagnosed infrequently. It is obvious from these data that the adjuvant chemotherapy of resected gastric cancer is of major interest—successful chemotherapy has the potential to improve long-term survival.

Single-Agent Studies

The Veterans Administration Surgical Oncology Group (VASOG) has been a pioneer in performing adjuvant studies in gastric cancer. Data from this group have shown that single-agent chemotherapy with thiothepa or fluorodeoxyuridine (FUdR) failed to improve 5-year disease-free survival. Of 194 patients randomized to receive thiothepa or no further treatment, 5-year survival was 25.5% vs 33.7%, and of 276 patients treated with FUdR vs no treatment, it was 23.9% vs 21.3%.[1,2]

Two-Drug Studies

During the mid-1970s three large randomized trials were initiated to assess the combination of 5-fluorouracil (5-FU) and methyl-CCNU. In the VASOG study 312 patients, 134 of whom had curative resections, were randomized between August 1974 and May 1980. For patients with complete resection median survival times in the treatment and control groups were similar: 27 months. Survival times at 3.5 years were 38.9% and 37.8%, respectively.

Patients with incomplete resections and nonresectable cases were also included in the trial. No differences were apparent between treatment and control groups in these patients as well: in those with incomplete resection the 1.5-year survival times were 29% and 31%, respectively. In unresectable cases median survival time was 6 months and 1-year survival, 13.9% and 14.7%, respectively.[3]

The Gastrointestinal Tumor Study Group (GITSG) randomized 142 patients with curative resections between January 1975 and September 1980. At a median follow-up of 4 years, median survival time in the treated group was significantly better than in the controls: 48+ months vs 33 months ($P<.03$).[4] The Eastern Cooperative Oncology Group (ECOG), however, conducted exactly the same trial from September 1975 to June 1980 and could not reproduce these positive results. Of 180 patients randomized, median survival time was 37 months in the treatment group and 33 months in the controls.[5] In a smaller German study encompassing 103 patients treated with 5-FU plus BCNU vs controls, no significant differences were observed between the two treatment arms.[6]

Cumulative data from these trials are depicted in Table 1. Although a strict comparison of these studies must be done with caution, these data strongly suggest that combining 5-FU with a nitrosourea is of no apparent benefit as an adjuvant treatment in patients with gastric carcinoma.

Combination Chemotherapy, Including Doxorubicin

Since the initial optimistic reports of combination chemotherapy including 5-FU (F), Adriamycin (A), and mitomycin C (FAM) in advanced disease,[7,8] several "third-generation" randomized studies have been initiated investigating this combination as an adjuvant treatment.

Preliminary results have been reported by the South West Oncology Group (SWOG) in 78 patients with no significant differences at a median follow-up of 2 years.[9] Employing the FAM regimen versus controls, the International Collaborative Cancer Group (ICCG) recently reported that of 286 fully evaluable

Table 1. Cumulative data of two-drug studies in resected gastric carcinoma[a]

Treatment group	Controls	Reference
36/66	36/68	b
29/71	40/71	c
57/91	51/89	d
10/44	17/54	e
132/272(49%)	144/282(51%)	

[a] Number of deaths/number of patients entered.
[b] Higgings GA, Amadeo JH, Smith DE, et al: Efficiency of prolonged intermittent therapy with combined 5-FU and methyl-CCNU following resection for gastric carcinoma. Cancer 1983;52:1105.
[c] The Gastrointestinal Tumor Study Group: Controlled trial of adjuvant chemotherapy following curative resection of gastric cancer. Cancer 1982;49:1116.
[d] Engstrom PF, Levin PT, Douglass HO, et al: Postoperative adjuvant 5-fluorouracil plus methyl-CCNU therapy for gastric cancer patients. Cancer 1985;55:1868.
[e] Schlag P, Schreml W, Gaus W, et al: Adjuvant 5-fluorouracil and BCNU chemotherapy in gastric cancer: 3-year results, in Recent Results in Cancer Research. Berlin-Heidelberg-New York, Springer, 1982, p 277.

patients after a median follow-up of 4 years, the mortality rate in the treatment arm was 45% vs 50% in the controls. Also, no significant differences were observed in subsets of patients with positive or negative nodes. Median survival in this study is expected to be 4 years for both treatment arms.[10] Other phase III studies of FAM vs controls, among them a study conducted by the Mid Atlantic Oncology Program (MAOP) and a trial initiated by the European Organization for Treatment and Cancer Research (EORTC) in 1981, are still in progress. In the EORTC trial 259 patients have been randomized, and the median survival of 185 evaluable patients is expected to be around 3.5 years. Considering the results published to date, it appears unlikely that a positive result will emerge from these studies.

The relatively long median survival time for all patients observed, especially in the ICCG and the EORTC studies compared with older trials, is of interest and underscores the value of randomized trials. A possible prolongation of survival is most likely the result of better preoperative staging with the use of CT scans.

Discussion

Since the initial report from Georgetown University (Washington, DC, USA) the FAM chemotherapy protocol has been adopted as "standard treatment" in advanced gastric cancer all over the world. Although the study conducted by the ECOG in advanced disease produced a 39% response rate for FAM and concluded that FAM should be strongly advocated for adjuvant treatment,[11] results of recent randomized trials have questioned the value of combination chemotherapy compared with 5-FU alone. Neither the North Central Cancer Treatment Group (NCCTG), which compared FAM with 5-FU,[12] nor an Italian study,[13] which compared FAM plus BCNU (BAFMI) with 5-FU, reported any differences in response rates[13] or survival times.[12,13]

A constant finding in all studies employing FAM, MeFA, or FAB has been the low complete response rate, mostly less than 5%. Chemotherapy protocols with such low complete response rates and overall response rates of around 30% (mostly excluding early deaths, toxic deaths, protocol violations, and losses to follow-up) are not likely to influence overall survival or benefit patients treated in an adjuvant setting.

Cisplatin has activity in gastric cancer and has therefore been added to FA (FAP). In six studies response rates have ranged between 29% and 59% and median survivals from 4 to 12 months. Some of these studies have reported a histologically documented complete response.[14] A further "new generation" regimen (EAP) comprises the combination of etoposide, Adriamycin, and cisplatin. A response rate of 72%, including some histologically documented complete responses, has been reported in 44 patients.[15] Finally, the combination of sequential high-dose MTX plus 5-FU combined with A (FAMTX), first published in 1982 with a response rate of 63%, was updated in 1986.[16] Of 100 patients, the 59 responses included 12 complete responses and a median survival time of 9 months. The EORTC GI Group has conducted a multicenter phase II study with this regimen and has reported 22 responders of 65 eligible patients including 9 complete responders, 3 of which were documented histologically.[17]

It is apparent that new treatment regimens, such as those discussed above, with a higher complete response rate and longer survival must be assessed further before adjuvant therapy can be expected to be worthwhile. It has been stated that new protocols should have a minimum response rate of 35% and a median survival time of greater than 7 months in phase II trials before being submitted to phase III testing.[18] Second-generation protocols such as FAP, EAP, and FAMTX are currently being tested by different groups in randomized trials and, it is hoped, will result in progress in the treatment of advanced gastric cancer. Only when this goal is achieved can adjuvant treatment be expected to yield positive results in resectable gastric cancer.

References

1. Dixon WJ, Longmire WP, Holden WD: Use of triethylenethiophosphoramide as an adjuvant to the surgical treatment of gastric and colorectal carcinoma: ten year follow up. Ann Surg 1971;173:16.
2. Serlin O, Wolkoff JS, Amadeo JH, et al: Use of 5-fluorodeoxyuridine (FudR) as an adjuvant to the surgical management of carcinoma of the stomach. Cancer 1969; 24:223.
3. Higgings GA, Amadeo JH, Smith DE, et al: Efficiency of prolonged intermittent therapy with combined 5-FU and methyl-CCNU following resection for gastric carcinoma. Cancer 1983;52:1105.
4. The Gastrointestinal Tumor Study Group: Controlled trial of adjuvant chemotherapy following curative resection of gastric cancer. Cancer 1982;49:1116.

5. Engstrom PF, Levin PT, Douglass HO, et al: Postoperative adjuvant 5-fluorouracil plus methyl-CCNU therapy for gastric cancer patients. Cancer 1985;55:1868.
6. Schlag P, Schreml W, Gaus W, et al: Adjuvant 5-fluorouracil and BCNU chemotherapy in gastric cancer: 3-year results, in Recent Results in Cancer Research. Berlin-Heidelberg-New York, Springer, 1982, p 277.
7. Macdonald JS, Schein PS, Woolley PV, et al: 5-Fluorouracil, doxorubicin and mitomycin C (FAM) combination chemotherapy for advanced gastric cancer. Ann Intern Med 1980;93:533.
8. Bitran JD, Desser RK, Kozloff MF, et al: Treatment of metastatic pancreatic and gastric adenocarcinoma with 5-fluorouracil, Adriamycin and mitomycin C (FAM). Cancer Treatm Rep 1979;63:2049.
9. Gagliano R, McCracken JD, Chen T: Adjuvant chemotherapy with 5-fluorouracil, Adriamycin and mitomycin (FAM) in gastric cancer—A SWOG study, abstract. Proc ASCO 1983;2:114.
10. Coombes RC, Schein PS, Chilvers C, et al: A controlled trial of FAM (5-FU, Adriamycin, mitomycin-C) chemotherapy as adjuvant treatment for resected gastric carcinoma, abstract. Cancer Chemother Pharmacol 1986;18(suppl 1):20.
11. Douglass HO, Lavin PT, Goudsmit A, et al: An Eastern Cooperative Oncology Group evaluation of combinations of methyl-CCNU, mitomycin-C, Adriamycin and 5-fluorouracil in advanced measurable gastric cancer (EST 2277). J Clin Oncol 1984;2:1372.
12. Cullinan SA, Moertel CG, Fleming TR, et al: A comparison of three chemotherapeutic regimens in the treatment of advanced pancreatic and gastric carcinoma. Fluorouracil vs fluorouracil and doxorubicin vs fluorouracil, doxorubicin and mitomycin. JAMA 1985;253:2061.
13. De Lisi V, Cocconi G, Tonato M, et al: Randomized comparison of 5-FU alone or combined with carmustine, doxorubicin and mitomycin (BAFMi) in the treatment of advanced gastric cancer. A phase III trial of the Italian Clinical Research Oncology Group (GOIRC). Cancer Treatm Rep 1986;70:481.
14. Wils J: Current status of chemotherapy for advanced gastric cancer. Anticancer Res 1987;7:755.
15. Preusser P, Wilke H, Achterrath W, et al: Advanced gastric carcinoma. A phase II study with etoposide (E), adriamycin (A) and split course cisplatin (P) = EAP, abstract. Proc ASCO 1987;6:75.
16. Klein HO, Dias Wickramanayake P, Farrokh G-H: 5-Fluorouracil (5-FU), adriamycin (ADM) and methotrexate (MTX)—a combination protocol (FAMTX) for treatment of metastasized stomach cancer, abstract. Proc ASCO 1986;5:84.
17. Wils J, Bleiberg H, Blijham G, et al: An EORTC gastrointestinal group evaluation of the combination of sequential methotrexate (MTX) and 5-fluorouracil (F), combined with adriamycin (A) (FAMTX) in advanced measurable gastric cancer. J Clin Oncol 1986;4:1799.
18. Killen JY, Ellenberg SS, Friedman MA: Combination chemotherapy (CT) regimens in advanced gastric cancer (GC), abstract. Proc ASCO 1985;4:82.

CHAPTER 13

Gastric Cancer Trials: Implications of the Gastrointestinal Tumor Study Group and the Mount Sinai Medical Center Experience

H.W. Bruckner

Introduction

The experience of the GITSG offers useful lessons. Physicians can avoid past "mistakes" and refine multidisciplinary treatment strategies of clear-cut therapeutic benefit. Trials had a sufficient number of patients to identify therapeutic manipulation which benefit a select minority. The sum of several manipulations, each of which may have limited applications, offers something for a substantial fraction of the patients in any physician's practice. As a consequence, it has become necessary to identify the unique features of the individual patient. This review will concentrate on the observations which are relevant to primary physicians, gastroenterologists, and surgeons.

There is an increasing need to evaluate and utilize additional now-important patient characteristics in data collection. This requires the efforts of pathologists, surgeons, and gastroenterologists, not only oncologists, in order to identify the optimum eligible patients for treatment with new strategies. Objective prognostic tests begin to predict risk of failure by site and may help to identify further treatment options for the increasing numbers of patients with apparent complete clinical remissions.

For early disease trials, optimum staging, earliest treatment, best supportive care (nutrition, pre/postoperative care), and adequate/increased dose-intensity (preferably of new drugs) may be critical for success. New regimens yield high complete response rates which satisfy the criteria for testing their use in adjuvant trials. Some patients with surgically reduced volume of regional disease and proven residual cancer survive 5 to 10 years without recurrent or progressive disease. This supports a selective role for coordinating debulking surgery with both radiotherapy and chemotherapy. New drugs offer opportunities for improving multidisciplinary management of operable and localized incompletely operable or inoperable stages of disease.

Advanced disease trials find that substitutes for MTC, such as MeCCNU, improve the tail of the survival curve, but not medial survival. Antifolates and cisplatin provide less toxic substitutes which further improve the tail of the survival curve. Some patients are already living longer as the result of attempting

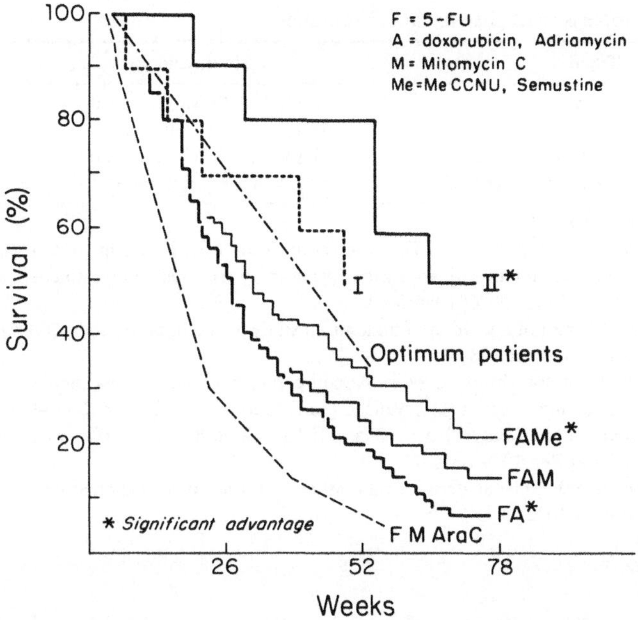

Fig. 1. The addition of new drugs to combination chemotherapy regimens has systematically improved survival: ADM (1975), MeCCNU (1979), CDDP and TZT (antifol). Optimum = entirely ambulatory, all laboratory tests (CBC, 6-12) normal.

these experimental options. Judicious use of experimental options may now offer a better chance of practical benefit for the majority of patients than so-called standard therapy.

Pilot studies, combining antifolates, CDDP, and biochemical modulation of 5-FU with LV, find an increased frequency of complete remission of far advanced disease. Complete remissions probably benefit the individual. Intensive new combination chemotherapy apparently offers more than a 50% chance of benefit for selected patients with advanced disease. This represents a milestone in creating new opportunities for multidisciplinary treatment strategies.

Advanced Disease

The GITSG series of controlled trials,[1-5] and other collaborative group trials are usually interpreted as evidence that chemotherapy has no impact on survival.[6] One can contend that this argument ignores some patients and evidence suggesting promising new experimental treatments which may potentially evolve into useful treatments. The survival curves differ "significantly" at 12 and 18 months, although they do not differ at the median of 6 months (Fig. 1). Mathematical models illustrate that some treatments prolong the survival of fewer than 35% of

Table 1. Comparison of gastric cancer regimens

Trend	Significant	Reference
FAT ≈ FAP > FAMe	(FAT/P > FAMe) Survival	a
FAMe > FAM > FA	(FAMe > FA) Survival	b
FAMe > FAM > FMeR > FMe	(FAMe > FMeR) Survival	c
FAMe > FAM > ADM > MFuCa	(ADM active) Response	d

R = Razoxane, ICRF 159.
[a] Bruckner HW, Stablein DM, for the Gastrointestinal Tumor Study Group: A randomized study of 5-fluorouracil and doxorubicin with semustine, cisplatin, or triazinate for treatment of advanced gastric cancer, abstract. Proc ASCO 1986;5:90.
[b] Gastrointestinal Tumor Study Group: Randomized study of combination chemotherapy in unresectable gastric cancer. Cancer 1984;53:13.
[c] Gastrointestinal Tumor Study Group: A comparative clinical assessment of combination chemotherapy in the management of advanced gastric carcinoma. *Cancer* 1982;49:1362.
[d] Gastrointestinal Tumor Study Group: Phase II-III chemotherapy studies in advanced gastric cancer. Cancer Treat Rep 1979;63:1871.
See also O'Connell MJ: Current status of chemotherapy for advanced pancreatic and gastric cancer. J Clin Oncol 1985;3:1032.

the patients without affecting the median (Bruckner, unpublished). The difference in the tail of the survival curve demonstrates improved quality of life for the "responding" patients. Treatment prolongs survival for these individuals. Best to worst treatments, as found by GITSG, are depicted in Table 1.

The interests of the few responding patients and the interests of the group do not conflict. Several drug regimens do have a substantial palliative benefit, but only for a few patients who are represented on the tail of the survival curves.

The well-intentioned concern that the large number who do not benefit are being hurt too much to justify benefiting the few who do respond is not supported by the data. Overall survival clearly does not suffer. No one seems ready to conduct a definitive trial of supportive care versus current best chemotherapy. Too few experienced physicians believe chemotherapy might lose in this trial.

Do these differences between treatments identify useful leads for the design of early disease trials? The survival differences become more substantive when applied to the GITSG regional disease trials.

The large number of trials constitutes a confirmatory meta-analysis. Real differences exist between treatments, which are applicable to subgroups. In identifying the subgroup, it is uncertain whether current assays predicting tumor sensitivity are of value, although assays would be if they could be improved. Their value would be in picking among the many sometimes active drugs.

With FAMe and FAM the toxicity of the long-acting agents can be catastrophic and limit their use in multidisciplinary therapy (radiotherapy) or adjuvant therapy. Schedule variations of these toxic drugs produced, at best, only small differences in the tail of survival curves.[7]

New drugs could be both less toxic and more effective than FAM. GITSG phase III trials have demonstrated the potential to break this toxicity barrier and to

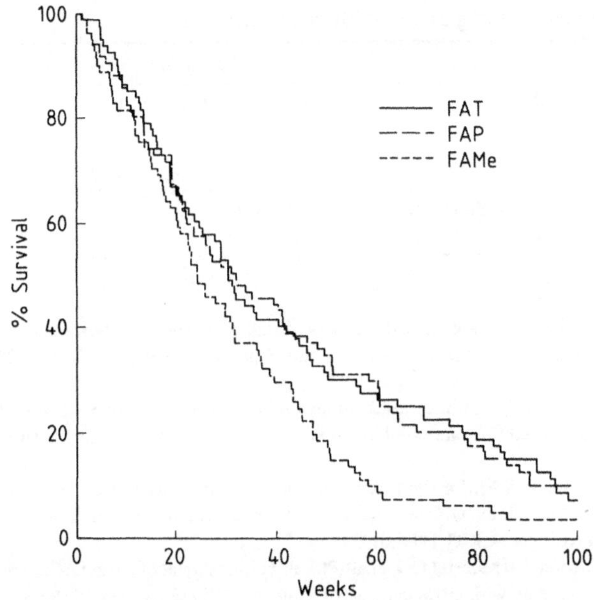

Fig. 2. Probability of survival by treatment. GITSG 8380.

improve the tail of the survival curve (Fig. 2). The GITSG most recent phase III study compared FAMe, FAP, and FAT, where P is cisplatin and T is the antifolate triazinate. For the first time, using either cisplatin or antifolate in combination chemotherapy can result in modestly better survival than with either FAM or FAMe.[5] The GITSG provides the most substantial phase III evidence to date that antifolates or CDDP advance safety and survival. This extends the highly promising and complementary response findings from the FA/MTX and EAP studies.[8-10] It is highly likely that phase III investigations of Klein and associates,[8] the EORTC investigators,[9] and Preusser and associates[10] will confirm these findings.

Trials using new drugs offer improved survival compared to regimens using standard drugs. This is entirely consistent with the numerous response-oriented phase II trials, especially of antifolates and cisplatin reviewed earlier in this symposium by Wils, Klein, and Preusser. The extensive body of phase II single-agent data favoring a role for CDDP was reviewed by Preusser and Wils today. Table 2 presents the series of GITSG trials identifying a role for TZT[4,5,11] alone and in combinations, confirmed by investigators from the Mayo Institute.[12]

Earlier GITSG studies of MTX alone[4] and MTX/5-FU at the Mount Sinai Medical Center[13] found evidence that MTX-produced objective tumor regression after standard 5-FU-containing therapy failed (Fig. 3). The GITSG MTX/5-FU[11] results included an apparent false-negative study.

Table 2A. Comparison of gastric cancer regimens: Triazinate

Trend	Significant	Reference
TZT > MTX > ICRF 159	(TZT > others) Survival	a
TZT phase II 2°	Response (?)	Unpublished
FAT < phase II (1°)	Survival	b
FAT > FAMe (1°)	(FAT > FAMe) Survival	c
FAT > FAMe (1°) renal dysfunction	Survival	c
MMC TZT phase II (2°)	Response	d

1° = primary therapy.
2° = secondary therapy.
[a] Bruckner HW, Lokich JJ, Stablein DM: Studies of Baker's antifol, methotrexate, and Razoxane in advanced gastric cancer. A Gastrointestinal Tumor Study Group Report. Cancer Treat Rep 1982; 66:1713.
[b] Bruckner HW, Stablein DM, for the Gastrointestinal Tumor Study Group: Single arm trials of triazinate, cisplatin and methotrexate combinations in advanced gastric cancer, abstract. Proc ASCO 1984;3:144.
[c] Bruckner HW, Stablein DM, for the Gastrointestinal Tumor Study Group: A randomized study of 5-fluorouracil and doxorubicin with semustine, cisplatin, or triazinate for treatment of advanced gastric cancer, abstract. Proc ASCO 1986;5:90.
[d] O'Connell MJ, Schutt AJ, Moertel CG, et al: Phase II clinical trial of triazinate in combination with mitomycin C for patients with advanced gastric cancer. J Clin Oncol 1987;5:83.

Table 2B. Comparison of gastric cancer regimens: Methotrexate

Regimen	Finding	Source
2° MTX low-dose	Response	GITSG
2° MTX[a] moderate-dose	Response	Mount Sinai
2° MTX[a] moderate-dose	Response failed	GITSG
2° MTX[b] moderate-dose	21% Response	Texas
1° MTX[a,b] high-dose	Response	Cologne
1° MTX[a,b] high-dose	Response	EORTC

1° = primary therapy.
2° = secondary therapy.
a = sequence with 5-FU.
b = sequence with ADM.

In extensively treated patients salvage therapy trials can fail yet prove misleading in that they represent false-negative findings. MTX alone had been active against gastric cancer on at least two occasions, therefore its total failure in the most recent trial may represent a false-negative.

Having demonstrated the activity of antifolates and CDDP in combination with 5-FU and ADM as doubling survival at 12 and 18 months,[5] the next Mount Sinai regimen "MLP" (Table 3) combined MTX/5-FU and LV/5-FU using the leucovorin both for rescue after the preceding MTX and potentiation of the subsequent 5-FU. LV is a cofactor that binds 5-fluoro-2-deoxyuridylate to thymidylate synthetase (TS), shown to double rates of response in three phase III colon cancer trials. It appears to act on all tested TS systems in vitro.[14] Machover and

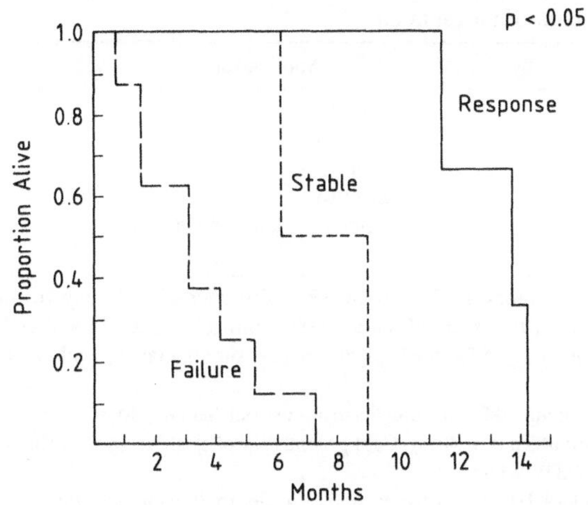

Fig. 3. Survival of patients with gastric carcinoma by response status from onset of therapy with a MTX/5-FU sequential regimen. All patients previously failed conventional regimens containing 5-FU and ADM such as FAM and MTX or FAMe with MeCCNU. (Reprinted with permission from Bruckner HW, Cohen J: MTX/5-FU trials in gastrointestinal and other cancers. Sem Oncol 1983;10:32.)

co-workers[15] found LV useful in gastric cancer testing 5-day loading schedule of daily LV/5-FU. However, Arbuck and co-workers,[16] testing a 6-week course of once weekly treatment, did not. These differences may be due to details of schedule, or the latter may be another example of a small false-negative trial. The decision to try to use LV/5-FU in the Mount Sinai regimen seems to be supported by the excellent findings with the etoposide/5-FU/LV trial for elderly patients presented today by Preusser. CDDP was added in conjunction with a 5-FU infusion. The infusion was considered preferable to bolus injections of 5-FU both because cisplatin is clearly synergistic with the infusion and because of some, as

Table 3. Mount Sinai MLP gastric cancer regimen: Schema for systemic treatment of gastric cancer

Hour	Drug	Dosage
0	MTX	160 → 200 → 300 mg/m²
4	5-FU	600 mg/m² (2nd time)
18	LV	200 mg/m²[a]
19	5-FU	600 mg/m²˙
19	5-FU Infusion	25 mg/kg/24 h × 96 h
20	CDDP	100 mg/m² with mannitol

Patients may be given MTX 160 mg/m² 0 time; 5-FU 500 mg/m² at 1 h, Days 1, 8 prior to starting this regimen, Day 15, to avoid delay for borderline postoperative recovery.
[a] LV 12.5 mg q6h × 4 days 2,9; double LV dosage, if complete gastrectomy or any high risks of toxicity due to MTX.

Table 4. MLP Mount Sinai regimen

Combination	Application	Reference
MTX/5-FU	Gastric	a,b
MTX/CDDP	In vitro	c
LV/5-FU	Colon, gastric	d
LV/5-FU/CDDP	In vitro	e
5-FU/CDDP	Clinical, adenoesophagus	e
CDDP/5-FU	Theoretical	–

[a] Klein HI, Dias Wichramanayake P, Farrokh GR: 5-Fluorouracil, adriamycin, and methotrexate—a combination protocol for treatment of metastasized stomach cancer. Proc ASCO 1986;5:84.
[b] Bruckner HW, Cohen J: MTX/5-FU trials in gastrointestinal and other cancers. Sem Oncol 1983;10:32.
[c] Bruckner HW, Stablein DM, for the Gastrointestinal Tumor Study Group: Sites of treatment failure: Gastrointestinal Tumor Study Group Analyses of gastric, pancreatic and colorectal trials. Cancer Treat Sym 1983;2:199.
[d] Arbuck SG, Douglass HO Jr, Trave F, et al: A phase II trial of 5-fluorouracil and high-dose intravenous leucovorin in gastric carcinoma. J Clin Oncol 1987;5:1150.
[e] Burchenal JH, Lokys L, Turkevich J, Gale G: Rationale of combination chemotherapy, in Prestayko AW, Crooke ST, Carter SK (eds): Cisplatin: Current Status and New Developments. New York, Academic Press, 1980, p 113.

yet unpublished, problems identified by GITSG in failing to deliver full doses of bolus 5-FU with simultaneous high doses of cisplatin.[5] These three regimens, compressed into 4 days, referred to as the MLP regimen in order to identify the novel components (MTX, LV, CDDP), actually represent five, possibly six, different potentially synergistic combinations. Cisplatin may be synergistic with LV/5-FU,[17] and MTX is sometimes highly synergistic with CDDP[18] (Table 4).

Five of the first ten patients have achieved complete remission with variations of this combination. The doses of the components were adjusted with the objective of giving as much as possible, enough to produce mild side effects, but reducing dosage to avoid risk of moderate or worse (nonhematologic side effects) on an individual basis.

These were all symptomatic, unusually sick, patients with larger than average, easily measurable, tumors. In addition, the speed of the response was perhaps unique to antifols. Complete responses sometimes occurred in only 4 to 8 weeks. We had sometimes observed this speed with the TZT regimen. Similar combinations are worthy of further testing. Complete responses with MLP and other regimens[8,9,10] will probably find a use in new treatment strategies and benefit the responding individual. MLP chemotherapy breaks a 50% benefit barrier for gastric cancer care. With eight of the first ten patients achieving partial or complete responses, at least half the treated patients now achieve some benefit from treatment.

The mild neurotoxicity of cisplatin may be limiting. Patients finally live long enough to risk cumulative toxicities. Gastric cancer may prove the first important indication for a less toxic cisplatin analogue. This is a priority for investigation in view of the multiple success of cisplatin against advanced gastric cancer and its predictable potential as a radiosensitizer for studies of regional disease.

Complete remissions create new clinical questions:

1. What is to be done once complete remission is achieved? Are these opportunities for biologic response modifiers, interleukin-2 radiotherapy, or surgery? The few residual cells have a far more rapid metabolism than the original bulk of the tumor if other tests of debulking with either chemotherapy or surgery apply. These active cells may in theory provide a rationale for testing schedule active drugs.

2. Are more precise and sensitive tests for residual disease necessary, and are they available? Will investigators need nuclear magnetic resonance imaging and new tumor markers, perhaps even more use of endoscopy and laparoscopy? The volume of residual tumors appears to be falling below the thresholds of computerized tomography and carcinoembryonic antigen assays.

3. What are the clinical and biological implications? Once frequent complete remissions are achieved, new sites of progression will appear. Formerly rare sites of progression, such as those in the central nervous system, increase in frequency of occurrence. It is time to reexamine sites of failure and reconsider the case for regional therapy of the stomach, peritoneum, or CNS if one site of progression proves predictably refractory to the new regimens. In the Mount Sinai experience, of the major gastrointestinal cancers, gastric cancer already demonstrates the greatest propensity to produce CNS carcinomatosis. Gastric cancers and the far more numerous colon cancers are equally likely to produce neurologic damage to the spine. The need to study the spine and prophylactic radiotherapy may become important. These implications need to be considered in planning both individual care and studies. They are not yet proven recommendations. Their importance, to quality of life, warrants bringing them to the clinician's early attention.

Time does not permit detailed discussion of clinical anecdotes. Some suggest a role for antiestrogen therapy, medroxyprogesterone or tamoxifen, in young women, especially those with a Krukenberg's tumor. The Krukenberg's tumor may represent an in vivo sensitivity test of hormonal dependence. Others suggest that increasing doses of MTX, from 160 to 300 to 600 mg/m^2, can be more effective, and that Ara-C, by biochemical-pharmacological criteria a good drug for intraperitoneal therapy and biochemical modulations, deserves evaluation in both IP therapy and sequential therapy.

The GITSG studies of natural history provide new information, sometimes refuting common clinical assumptions.[19-21] Gastric cancer is a systemic disease. No one site of metastasis kills enough patients to warrant tests of regional therapy except possibly the stomach itself.[19] Investigators must first find a subpopulation (if any exists) eligible for such studies. Regional therapy trials are not rational for any large fractions of patients (based on a failure to find any relationship between one site of metastatic disease and survival; in addition, the severity of regional disease probably must be graded [1 to 5+] based on both degree of

Table 5. Intraperitoneal overflow therapy: Advantages and goals

Allows best duplication of laboratory conditions (concentration × time)
Maximum dosage
Maximum duration
Least systemic toxicity
Also serves as systemic therapy
Suitable for *large tumors*
No delay in *systemic therapy*

disease and severity of consequences if studies of regional disease and its therapy are to be interpretable [Bruckner, manuscript in preparation]).

Overflow IP therapy, as developed at the Mount Sinai Medical Center (Table 5), represents a way to test IP therapy. Systemic therapy cannot be delayed or dosage compromised in order to investigate IP therapy because gastric cancer is a rapidly fatal systemic disease. By creating deliberate overflow the clinician can give sufficiently large IP dosages to achieve simultaneous full-strength systemic therapy. Symptomatic patients do benefit from intraperitoneally administered MTX/5-FU, LV/5-FU, and CDDP/5-FU as tested here in several schedules (Table 6). Unfortunately, without controls, failing the same systemic therapy, it is uncertain whether the route and greater IP concentration of drugs, or simply the choice of drugs, is responsible for the benefit.

Clinical impressions are often misleading. Physicians are sometimes too pessimistic—the spectrum of survival is more heterogeneous than they appreciate. Size of tumor and number of involved organs influence prognosis, but biochemical tests and complete blood count abnormalities are the major prognostic determinants.[20,21,22] Large tumors with normal laboratory tests are much less serious than small tumors with even subtly abnormal laboratory tests.[22] Rates of response may be directly related to prognostic factors.[20]

One can make a case for early treatment before the patient becomes symptomatic or laboratory tests change for the worse. The risk of complications of therapy is also less. Sometimes chemotherapy will only stabilize disease. It is better

Table 6. Intraperitoneal regimens

Drug	mg/m²	Time	Drug	mg/m²	Time
MTX	200–400	0 h	MTX	200–400	0 h
5-FU	1000	2 h	5-FU	1000	2 h
LV	100–200	3 h			
CDDP	100	4 h	LV	100–200	18 h
			&	10 q6×3	
			IV not PO 5-FU	1000	19h
			CDDP	100	20 h

Compare early vs late treatment 2, 3, 4 vs 2, 18, 19, 20.
First time 2, 3, 4, then if tolerated → 2, 18, 19, 20.

Table 7. Possible new approaches to obstructing gastric lesions

Laser endoscopy preferred to prosthesis, which creates too many complications.
Simultaneous radiotherapy-chemotherapy preferred to surgery for patients with a poor prognosis; later surgery for complete responders; stents for nonresponders.
Acute parenteral nutrition (normal, not hypercaloric) preferred to waiting for failure of oral feeding, waiting at the cost of serious nutritional and immunological deficiencies.

to treat early and stabilize asymptomatic disease rather than to delay and only stabilize, thereby suspending some patient with refractory symptoms.

Prognostic tests may also help demonstrate objective criteria for surgery by testing their relation to outcome. Promising candidate tests include the GITSG objective chemistry and hematology tests, immunology profiles, measures of tumor diploidy, and perhaps single-dose, in vivo, chemotherapy sensitivity tests. When does it pay either to debulk surgically or give preoperative combined modality therapy? Testing putative prognostic factors may assist in selecting among these options. Patients with poor prognostic profiles can probably be better managed without exploration or surgery; these need rapid uncomplicated evaluation and systemic treatment, using the laser to correct or prevent obstruction. The Mount Sinai experience finds that prosthetic tubes complicate future care, and even follow-up tests, without providing true relief of obstruction (Table 7). A combination of laser surgery and radio- and chemotherapy for local control is a testable alternative to either the tube or even surgery, especially now that rates of response with systemic treatment and radiosensitizers have improved. The broad conclusions and implications for conduct of new advanced disease trials are presented in Tables 8 and 9.

Regional Therapy

Findings of the GITSG trials suggest that the benefit of treatment for regional disease is far different from that of the identical treatment for metastatic disease.[23]

Table 8. Findings of advanced gastric cancer trials

1. 30% Rates of complete response with antifolates or cisplatin MTX/5-FU, ADM, EAP
2. Both individually double survival at 1 year 30% vs 15%; FAT or FAP vs FAMe, (GITSG)
3. Compared with 1 and 2 above, MTX/5-FU, LV/5-FU, and CDDP/5-FU infusion can be combined in a 4-day regimen (Mount Sinai); this tends to increase both complete and partial response rates further
4. Anecdotal experience suggests the need for:
   i. More sensitive follow-up tests (tumor marker assays, laparoscopy, endoscopy, NMR)
   ii. A less neurotoxic CDDP regimen
   iii. MTX dose–response studies
   iv. Evaluation of antiestrogens (Krukenberg's tumors)
   v. Evaluation of Ara-C (regional therapy) and biochemical modulation

Table 9. Modifications of advanced gastric cancer trials

More than 50% of patients can be expected to achieve some objective response with clinical benefit. Complete response goals create requirements for:

i. Natural history and prognostic studies
ii. Better follow-up tests to measure initial and residual tumor
iii. Less initial, more selective, surgery; early start of chemotherapy; no longer delay systemic therapy, for surgery in some cases, not even for gastric obstruction (Table 7)
iv. Emphasis on achievement of complete response, not maintenance of partial responses
v. Sequential therapy with complete response and its consolidation as the new objectives
vi. Prospective studies of site-definite risk and feasibility of specific sites of failure (stomach, peritoneum, liver, meninges)

Several regimens (FAT, FAP > FAMe) improve the tail of the survival curve. New regimens (MLP > EAP > FAMTX) may improve median survival as well, if phase II findings are reproducible

Objective prognostication from CBC/12 possible.

Survival, when disease is limited to the potential radiotherapy field, is more clearly influenced by (even) the last generation of treatment options. Some patients may be cured. Individual differences in details of chemotherapy (timing, choice of drugs) and debulking apparently make a much greater difference in treatment of regional than of metastatic disease. In GITSG randomized studies, stratified for stage (regional versus advanced), differences were found in median

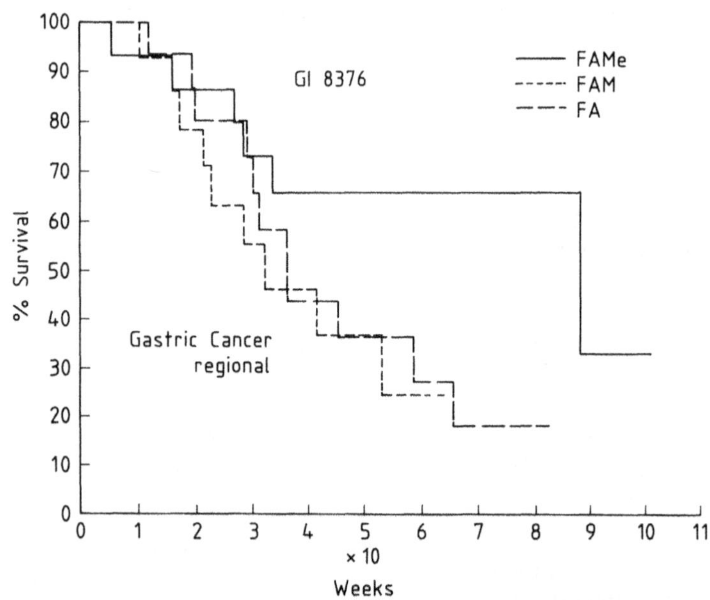

Fig. 4. Survival of a subset of randomized patients with localized inoperable residual gastric cancer.

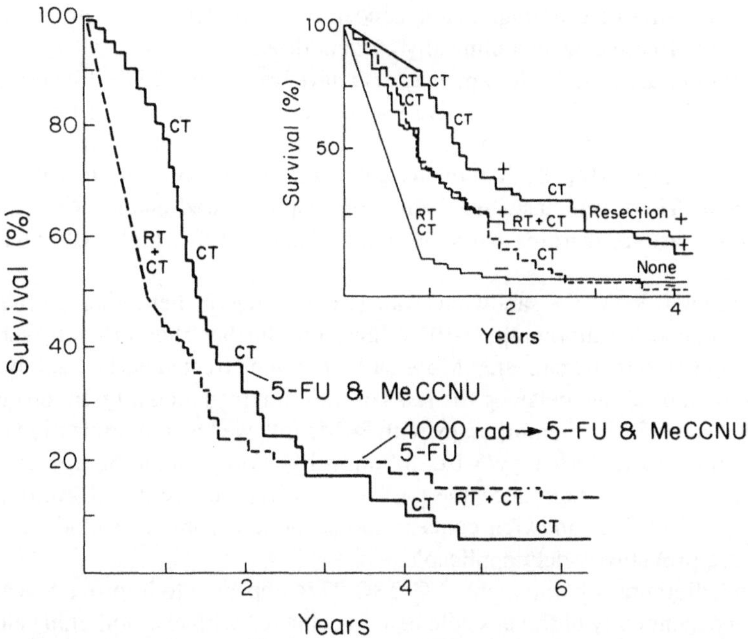

Fig. 5. Chemotherapy delays distant recurrence and prolongs survival; radiotherapy possibly increases 5-year survival (nonsignificant); palliative resection of the primary tumor increases median and 5-year survival. (Reprinted with permission from Gastrointestinal Tumor Study Group: A comparison of combination chemotherapy and combined modality for locally advanced gastric carcinoma. Cancer 1982;49:1771.)

survival of patients with regional disease, while in the group with advanced disease differences were found only in comparing the tail of the survival curves (GITSG, unpublished observations; references 2, 3). For patients with regional disease, who represent a randomized subgroup of early GITSG (collected) advanced disease trials, the individual addition of some drugs is clearly beneficial, albeit only palliative. For example, adding Wednesday, July 13, 1988ADM results in FAMe, which is superior to FMe; as a substitute, MeCCNU (FAMe) is superior to MTX (FAM). An apparently ineffective drug may have a demonstrable role in regional or in theory even adjuvant therapy (Bruckner and Stablein, in preparation) (Fig. 4).

The GITSG 8274 trial (Fig. 5) found an advantage for chemotherapy (FMe) reflected in improved 25th–50th percentile survival, and also a small, statistically significant advantage for radiotherapy at 4 to 5 years. The survival curves crossed. Both chemotherapy and radiotherapy apparently benefit different requirements of gastric cancer patients with regional disease.[24]

Delays in starting chemotherapy may have led to early (fatal) progression of occult systemic metastases.[23] 5-FU infusion also delays the appearance of occult, usually non-life-threatening, colon cancer in phase III trials, although it is minimally effective against clinically evident disease.[25]

Premature use of radiotherapy may also have been toxic. GITSG investigators were unable to identify the relative role of poor nutrition, site of progression, treatment-related toxicity, and the tumor itself to the early fatalities. Exact mechanism of (early) death remains unknown, even those due to cancer, not treatment. There remains a need for more sophisticated quantitative descriptive information regarding pathophysiologic mechanism which may impact on survival.

These trials led to the sandwich strategy consisting of chemotherapy followed by simultaneous radiotherapy/5-FU followed by further chemotherapy successfully applied to rectal cancer.[26] More patients can be treated earlier, safely, with chemotherapy alone, delaying the risks of the combined modality. In the current GITSG trial (8380), chemotherapy with FAMe followed by randomization of half the patients to radiotherapy/5-FU followed by FAMe chemotherapy confirms that therapists can reproduce the past early palliative result and avoid excess early toxicity. The sandwich concept and sequential combined modality treatment are probably widely applicable.

The radiotherapy component of GITSG 8274 appeared to improve 5-year survival independently of the possible benefit achieved with chemotherapy alone.[24] This needs to be confirmed. In the case of regional disease there are multiple examples of radiotherapy with simultaneous 5-FU, but not of radiotherapy alone, improving the tail of the survival curve. Sometimes the combined modality even improved 5-year survival (Table 10). There are numerous other examples relevant to gastrointestinal cancer: in pancreatic cancer[27,28]; in rectal cancer[26,29]; and possibly others[30,31]; for anal cancer the examples are too numerous to cite. Nevertheless, in the specific 8274 study, chemotherapy alone appears to produce

Table 10. Gastric cancer: Radiotherapy and 5-FU

High local failure rates, historically problematic in GITSG
More extensive surgery associated with increased morbidity
RT/5-FU vs RT, double-blind, survival[a]
RT/5-FU vs 5-FU/MeCCNU[b]
5-year survivors despite initial proven residual disease; RT/5-FU appears superior to CT
Median survival advantage of chemotherapy
Sandwich 5-FU/MeCCNU → RT/5-FU → 5-FU/MeCCNU in progress[c]
5-FU infusion ± RT, small (2 cm) lesions medically inoperable[d]
2 of 2 complete remissions without surgery 1+ year

[a] Moertel CG, Childs DS, Reitemeirer RJ, et al: Combined 5-fluorouracil and supervoltage radiation therapy of locally unresectable gastrointestinal cancer. Lancet 1969;2:865.
[b] Gastrointestinal Tumor Study Group: A comparison of combination chemotherapy and combined modality for locally advanced gastric carcinoma. Cancer 1982;149:1771.
[c] GITSG, unpublished.
[d] Bruckner HW: Letter to the Editor. Am J Gastroenterol, to be published.

Table 11. Regional gastric cancer trials

1. Debulking is palliative, possibly curative (needs to be confirmed) (GITSG, Japan).
2. Adjuvant, radiotherapy-chemotherapy probably cures ≈20% of the debulked patients (GITSG).
3. Chemotherapy is demonstrably palliative (GITSG).
4. Radiotherapy is controversial but "probably" curative for 5% to 10% of patients (GITSG).
5. Need more detailed data collection regarding site of failure; cause of death; supportive care; nutrition (GITSG).
6. Periadjuvant chemotherapy-radiotherapy can "sterilize" small disease in medically inoperable patients (Mount Sinai).
7. Models begin to favor preoperative treatment, CT→ ±CT-RT → ±surgery → CT, with selective surgery at decision point.

5-year survivors, although less often than does the combined modality.[24] The observed impact on survival achieved with chemotherapy or chemotherapy-radiotherapy establishes the need for definitive studies with superior radiosensitizers such as 5-FU infusion with cisplatin and combination regimens which produce high rates of complete response.

The GITSG experience demonstrated the need to debulk the patient in order to achieve best results with the weak regimens then available.[24] Nevertheless one cannot conclude which strategy, pre- or postoperative treatment, would be the current optimum. As described by Klein and Preusser at this symposium, new and more potent chemotherapy may frequently produce high quality debulking before either radiotherapy or surgery. In theory, the new chemotherapy may be competitive with debulking surgery because it also provides: (1) earlier systemic treatment, (2) no loss of patients due to surgical morbidity, and (3) an in vivo sensitivity test.

In this conference Klein, Wils, and Preusser agree that it is sometimes possible to eradicate regional disease. It is hoped that these more potent regimens will improve further upon GITSG success with less intensive regimens, which already produce some 5-year survivors. In planning treatment for regional gastric cancer, the issue is cure—not merely palliation. Of interest, serendipity provided the opportunity to treat medically inoperable early gastric cancer. These sometimes can be rendered complete remissions with much less intensive therapy, further support for testing the new regimens.[32]

Japanese studies provide both a supporting and cautionary observation. They support palliative debulking. Some patients with positive margins survive without further therapy.[33] This also establishes the need for more thorough description of residual disease to insure that "cures" can be correctly attributed to additional therapy. Some GITSG survivors had more than microscopic residual disease, suggesting therapy contributed to the cures.[23]

The conclusions and implications of these studies are summarized in Tables 11 and 12.

Table 12. Modifications of regional therapy of gastric cancer

Top priority for cure as a study goal; potential for cure with combined modality, combination chemotherapy and possibly even with debulking surgery alone
Potent regimens create promising testable alternatives to debulking unresectable tumor with surgery i. Debulking with more potent drug combinations; then, if needed, simultaneous chemotherapy-radiotherapy before surgery ii. Extend preoperative treatment to intermediate-sized tumors; there are already anecdotal CRp's with mild regimens
Primary tumors may be more sensitive to chemotherapy than metastatic tumor; change of a single agent in chemotherapeutic regimen may substantially improve median survival, even drugs failing in advanced disease trials. Assessment of drug effect on the primary tumor is a potentially useful guide to order of comprehensive therapy.

CRp = pathologically proven complete response.

Adjuvant Therapy

The GITSG adjuvant trial comparing 5-FU and MeCCNU versus observations after curative resection stands almost alone in finding a survival benefit of 15% to 25% associated with the use of adjuvant chemotherapy (Fig. 6).[34] This apparent benefit attributable to chemotherapy was found in every subgroup defined by nodal status (positive or negative) and surgery (subtotal versus total) or primary site (distal versus proximal) (Fig. 6). There is no clear answer as to why one trial succeeded when others failed. There is a less than 5% likelihood for them to be false-successes, because of the nature of the statistical tests. In contrast, small trials have a 20% to 40% risk of false-failure to detect 10% to 20% survival differences between treatments (power issues). There is a clear precedent in the colon adjuvant trials. Small trials with similar MeCCNU-vincristine-5-FU (MOF) regimens apparently failed, but, in contrast, a 1000 patient trial was clearly successful.[30,31] Perhaps the size of future gastric cancer adjuvant trials should be larger to provide more realistic tests. On the other hand, two of the GITSG members (Mount Sinai Medical Center and Mayo Clinic) individually succeeded in finding statistically demonstrable benefit with treatment as part of the GITSG 8174 trial. The two substudies further support the evidence of benefit due to treatment.

Perhaps these institutions at the time were the largest and most experienced contributors and were especially rigorous in pathology review. Clinicians made many errors in understaging due to reliance on routine pathology reports and lack of assistance from the surgeons in describing the orientation and margins of the specimen. Gastric tumors have three-dimensional margins.[35] They interface with the omentum, spleen, and pancreas, not only with the proximal and distal gut. The GITSG examined several possible explanations for its success in a trial which others failed to reproduce.[36] Unfortunately, data from the other trials are not available in a form which provides for testing. This demonstrated the need to address several issues fully in the future.[36,37] Based on the aforementioned qual-

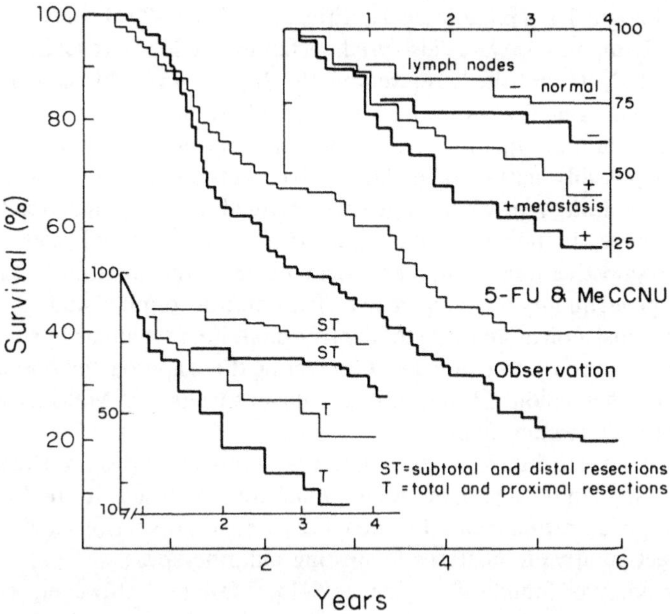

Fig. 6. Chemotherapy increases survival in every subset after potentially curative resection, especially patients with metastases in resected lymph nodes and/or proximal primary tumors. GITSG 8174. (Reprinted with permission from Douglass HO, Stablein D, Bruckner HW, et al: Controlled trial of adjuvant chemotherapy following curative resection for gastric cancer. Cancer 1982;49:1116.)

ity of staging, the GITSG 8174 trial may have had fewer ineligible patients, because inappropriate referrals were excluded. The GITSG may also have started treatment earlier with less delay after surgery.

Early start of adjuvant therapy in some clinical situations is almost a prerequisite for success.[37] In animal models, the remaining tumor is more susceptible to chemotherapy only in a brief postsurgical period. Japanese gastric cancer trials which find benefit for adjuvant therapy may also have started treatment earlier than those which failed.[36,37]

The GITSG may have given more medicine, more intensively. Adequate dose intensity, because of the steep nature of the dose–response curves, is probably critical to success. Inadequate dosage provides an inadequate test of therapy. Unlike 10 years ago, many more physicians are willing to give early intensive therapy. Adjuvant trials are especially susceptible to multiple seemingly little but actually consequential mistakes.

There is no evidence that past gastric cancer adjuvant trials harmed the patients.[35] Treatment is not associated with an inferior survival pattern. Trials 8174 and 8180 demonstrate the value and reliability of the stratification variables. Proximal tumors are clearly worse than distal tumors. They are probably separate etiological and pathological entities, based on GITSG analyses of site of failure.[19,28] Lymph-node status also predicts failure (as does serosal involvement) (Douglass et al, unpublished; references 19, 28, 35, 36). This is analogous to demonstrations using the Astler Coller Staging System.

Application of more quantitative details—number of nodes, level of involved nodes, and possibly nature of nodal involvement—microscopic, whether the architecture is destroyed, whether grossly enlarged, nature of reaction (invasion by lymphocytes, monocytes, and natural killer cells)—could lead to highly accurate prognostication. Computer assistance opens the possibility of a heretofore unimagined quality of matched historical controls for pilot studies, provided one does not insist on attempting to identify small improvements in survival due to treatment. There is some precedent for testing these approaches based on both GITSG and other colon[30,31] and gastric adjuvant trials.[35,36] Multivariate prognostication is quite consistent.

Analysis of sites of failure assists in selecting future priorities for investigation, and identifying suitable patients for regional therapy trials. It allows a test of whether there is a rational case for the more extensive operations and may identify or reject putative indications for testing radiotherapy.

Initially, analyses found little evidence of local failure.[19] However, the GITSG improved its reporting by emphasizing this question. There may be a trend identifying the stomach as a site of recurrence. However, even now it is uncertain whether there is enough isolated local recurrence as opposed to simultaneous sites of failure in the stomach to warrant adjuvant treatment of the stomach and surrounding drainage areas. Perhaps 30% to 50% of tumors will recur locally. Statistically, this is frequent enough to warrant trials designed to prevent regional recurrence. However, initial analyses found that gastric cancer recurred in multiple sites: most frequently in liver, then peritoneum, then bone.[19] Nor is it certain that the local recurrence is a sufficiently common cause of morbidity or mortality to allow trial methods. This is particularly true of the proximal junction cancers.[19] The distal cancers might have more local recurrences without concurrent distant disease, but the lesson is that GITSG investigations are having trouble proving that any subgroup of patients is suitable for trials designed to prevent local recurrence. Nevertheless, the intraperitoneal overflow concept may lend itself to adjuvant therapy.[35,36] Investigators must first identify the ideal group of patients for this study rather than simply risk a large adjuvant-regional therapy study. This caveat is strengthened in that the new more potent regimens may decrease the need for any regional therapy. Systemic treatment has priority for investigation.

Analyses of prognostic factors associated with recurrence can identify a group of patients with sufficiently high risk of failure to justify trials of the most successful new intensive chemotherapy regimens. As an adjuvant treatment they will probably be palliative for half the patients, as they appear to be for patients with metastatic disease. There is a limited precedent in breast cancer adjuvant trials. First studies targeted the subgroup with the highest risk of recurrence. The recent success of systemic therapy for advanced gastric cancer and combined modality therapy for regional gastric cancer implies opportunities for successful adjuvant therapy, because in adjuvant therapy the occult tumor burden is substantially smaller than the advanced primary tumors now successfully irradicated.

The several successful demonstrations that intensive chemotherapy produces 30% or more complete remissions should encourage preoperative trials (effectively an attempt at in vivo sensitivity testing) before surgery.

Chemotherapy may sometimes be followed by chemotherapy plus simultaneous radiotherapy before definitive surgery.

Contrary to current practice goals, patients with intermediately sized tumors are the most likely beneficiaries of adjuvant therapy, including preoperative regional therapy. This premise is based on mathematical models in part derived from successful regional therapy for anal cancer (Bruckner, manuscript in preparation). The smallest tumors provide too little risk for statistical tests. The largest tumors are too often already subclinically metastatic or too large for local control. Only tumors of intermediate size appear to have the optimum balance of risk and feasibility of effective therapy.

The GITSG adjuvant trial 8180 compared 5-FU and MeCCNU (FMe) with or without ADM as adjuvant therapy. Preliminary survival curves suggest this trial may reproduce past GITSG findings of GITSG trial 8174. This, however, would not serve to confirm the efficacy of adjuvant therapy. The database is insufficient to test for cross-trial overall differences of even 20% in survival although they would be clinically substantial. The trial was closed prematurely. Chemotherapists are less and less enthusiastic about ADM, although ADM alone produces tumor regression as frequently as any single drug tested against gastric cancer. The low response rates achieved with ADM alone and the even lower dosage used in combination chemotherapy regimens also suggest this trial will fail. This is especially true if the two-drug control regimen has any efficacy in some of the same population which responds to ADM, because it will blunt any possible differences. In theory, ultra-high dose ADM alone is of more interest than FAM or FAMe but of less interest than novel combinations.

Table 13. Modifications of adjuvant therapy

A. (As complete response rates increase, effective chemotherapy creates realistic *testable* options which offer more hope than standard therapy for the majority of patients.)

Define risk-intensity subgroups for adjuvant studies:

i. Good (low-recurrence) risk for tests of biological response modifiers
ii. Poor risk for tests of intensive chemotherapy near certain occult metastases
iii. High risk of regional relapse for tests of regional therapy
Combine CT with RT preoperatively for small tumors vs postoperatively for large tumors vs before and after for largest tumors

Preoperative in vivo sensitivity testing for intensive adjuvant therapy (if therapy produces CRp, it follows some must benefit from adjuvant therapy).

CRp = pathologically proven complete remission.

Table 14. Recommended modifications of adjuvant gastric cancer studies

A.	Increase detail of prospective surgery and pathology records to improve identification of patients with *low risk* of isolated local failure ineligible for extended surgery or combined modality therapy
B.	More active combinations produce 30% complete response; FAM and FAMe do not satisfy criteria of an adjuvant regimen
C.	More intensive treatments avoid suboptimum part of the dose-response curve
D.	Earlier start of adjuvant treatment
E.	Increase size of studies to detect the expected 25% frequency of benefit

The new cisplatin and antifol regimens described today by several groups of investigators appear to create an entirely better opportunity for adjuvant chemotherapy. By any rationale criteria, the FMe, FAMe, and FAM generation of regimens has been brushed aside by the potential advantages of these new regimens (Tables 13 and 14).

References

1. Gastrointestinal Tumor Study Group: Phase II-III chemotherapy studies in advanced gastric cancer. Cancer Treat Rep 1979;63:1871.
2. Gastrointestinal Tumor Study Group: A comparative clinical assessment of combination chemotherapy in the management of advanced gastric carcinoma. Cancer 1982;49:1362.
3. Gastrointestinal Tumor Study Group: Randomized study of combination chemotherapy in unresectable gastric cancer. Cancer 1984;53:13.
4. Bruckner HW, Lokich JJ, Stablein DM: Studies of Baker's antifol, methotrexate, and Razoxane in advanced gastric cancer. A Gastrointestinal Tumor Study Group Report. Cancer Treat Rep 1982;66:1713.
5. Bruckner HW, Stablein DM, for the Gastrointestinal Tumor Study Group: A randomized study of 5-fluorouracil and doxorubicin with semustine, cisplatin, or triazinate for treatment of advanced gastric cancer, abstract. Proc ASCO 1986;5:90.
6. O'Connell MJ: Current status of chemotherapy for advanced pancreatic and gastric cancer. J Clin Oncol 1985;3:1032.
7. Douglass HO Jr, Lavin PT, Goudsmit A, et al: An Eastern Cooperative Oncology Group evaluation of combinations of methyl-CCNU, mitomycin-C, Adriamycin, and 5-fluorouracil in advanced measurable gastric cancer (EST 2277). J Clin Oncol 1984;2:1372.
8. Klein HI, Dias Wichramanayake P, Farrokh GR: 5-Fluorouracil, Adriamycin, and methotrexate – a combination protocol for treatment of metastasized stomach cancer. Proc ASCO 1986;5:84.
9. Wils J, Bleiberg H, Dalesio O, et al: An EORTC gastrointestinal group evaluation of the combination of sequential methotrexate and 5-fluorouracil, combined with Adriamycin in advanced measurable gastric cancer. J Clin Oncol 1986;4:1799.
10. Preusser P, Wilke H, Achterrath W, et al: Advanced gastric carcinoma: A phase II study with etoposide, Adriamycin and split course cisplatin. Proc ASCO 1987;6:75.

11. Bruckner HW, Stablein DM, for the Gastrointestinal Tumor Study Group: Single arm trials of triazinate, cisplatin and methotrexate combinations in advanced gastric cancer, abstract. Proc ASCO 1984;3:144.
12. O'Connell MJ, Schutt AJ, Moertel CG, et al: Phase II clinical trial of triazinate in combination with mitomycin C for patients with advanced gastric cancer. J Clin Oncol 1987;5:83.
13. Bruckner HW, Cohen J: MTX/5-FU trials in gastrointestinal and other cancers. Sem Oncol 1983;10:32.
14. Houghton JA, Houghton PJ: Basis for the interaction of 5-fluorouracil and leucovorin in colon adenocarcinoma, in Bruckner HW, Rustum YM (eds): Advances in Cancer Chemotherapy: The Current Status of 5-Fluorouracil-Leucovorin Calcium Combination. New York, Park Row, 1984, p 23.
15. Machover D, Schwarzenberg L, Goldschmidt E, et al: Treatment of advanced colorectal and gastric adenocarcinomas with 5-FU combined with high-dose folinic acid: a pilot study. Cancer Treat Rep 1982;66:1803.
16. Arbuck SG, Douglass HO Jr, Trave F, et al: A phase II trial of 5-fluorouracil and high-dose intravenous leucovorin in gastric carcinoma. J Clin Oncol 1987;5:1150.
17. Trave F, Rustum YM, Goranson J: Synergistic antitumor activity of cisplatin and 5-fluorouracil in mice bearing leukemia L1210 cells, abstract. Proc ASCO 1985;26:322.
18. Burchenal JH, Lokys L, Turkevich J, et al: Rationale of combination chemotherapy, in Prestayko AW, Crooke ST, Carter SK (eds): Cisplatin: Current Status and New Developments. New York, Academic Press, 1980, p 113.
19. Bruckner HW, Stablein DM, for the Gastrointestinal Tumor Study Group: Sites of treatment failure: Gastrointestinal Tumor Study Group Analyses of gastric, pancreatic and colorectal trials. Cancer Treat Sym 1983;2:199.
20. Lavin PT, Bruckner HW, Plaxe SC, for the Gastrointestinal Tumor Study Group: Studies in prognostic factors relating to chemotherapy for advanced gastric cancer. Cancer 1983;50:2016.
21. Bruckner HW, Lavin P, Plaxe S, et al: Routine clinical chemistries as improved determinates of prognosis for patients with metastatic cancer of the stomach. Oncology1983;40:31.
22. Bruckner HW, Lavin PT, Plaxe SC, et al: Absolute granulocyte, lymphocyte and monocyte counts. Useful determinants of prognosis for patients with metastatic cancer of the stomach. JAMA 1982;247:1004.
23. Gastrointestinal Tumor Study Group: A comparison of combination chemotherapy and combined modality for locally advanced gastric carcinoma. Cancer 1982;49:1771.
24. Stablein DM, Carter WH, et al: Analysis of survival data with nonproportional hazard functions. Control Clin Trials 1981;2:149.
25. Kemeny N, Daly J, Reichman B, et al: Intrahepatic or systemic infusion of fluorodeoxyuridine in patient with liver metastases from colorectal carcinoma. Ann Intern Med 1987;107:459.
26. Krook J, Moertel C, Wieand H, et al: Radiation vs sequential chemotherapy-radiation-chemotherapy. A study of the North Central Cancer Treatment Group, Duke University, and the Mayo Clinic. Proc ASCO 1986;5:82.
27. Moertel CG, Childs DS, Reitemeirer RJ, et al: Combined 5-fluorouracil and supervoltage radiation therapy of locally unresectable gastrointestinal cancer. Lancet 1969;2:865.

28. Gastrointestinal Tumor Study Group: A multi-institutional comparative trial of radiation therapy alone and in combination with 5-fluorouracil for locally unresectable pancreatic carcinoma. Ann Surg 1979;189:126.
29. Gastrointestinal Tumor Study Group: Prolongation of the disease-free interval in surgically treated rectal carcinoma. N Engl J Med 1985;312:1465.
30. Wolmark N, Fisher B, Rockette H, et al: Adjuvant therapy in carcinoma of the colon: five year results of NSABP protocol C-01. Proc ASCO 1987;6:92.
31. Fisher B, Wolmark N, Rockette H, et al: Adjuvant chemotherapy or post-operative radiation for rectal cancer: 5-year results of NSABP R-01. Proc ASCO 1987;6:92.
32. Bruckner HW: Letter to the Editor. Am J Gastroenterol, to be published.
33. Nakazato H, Imanaga H: Results of surgery for gastric cancer and effect of adjuvant chemotherapy, in Herfarth Ch, Schlag P (eds): Gastric Cancer. Berlin-Heidelberg-New York, Springer, 1979, p 344.
34. Douglass HO, Stablein D, Bruckner HW, et al: Controlled trial of adjuvant chemotherapy following curative resection for gastric cancer. Cancer 1982;49:1116.
35. Kabakow B, Storch JA, Bruckner HW: New multidisciplinary treatment for gastric carcinoma. Digestion 1977;16:248.
36. Douglass HO Jr: Western surgical adjuvant trials in gastric cancers: lessons from current trials to be applied to the future, in: Contemporary Issues in Clinical Oncology. New York, Churchill-Livingston, 1988, p 145.
37. Douglass HO Jr: Adjuvant chemotherapy-stomach cancer-adjuvant treatment of gastric cancer, in: Cancer Chemotherapy: Challenges for the Future. First Nagoya Intern Symp on Cancer Treatment. Excerpta Medica International Congress Series 729, 1985.

CHAPTER 14

Preoperative ("Neoadjuvant") Chemotherapy in Locally Advanced Gastric Carcinoma

H. Wilke, P. Preusser, U. Fink, W. Achterrath, H.-J. Meyer, H.J. Schmoll, and H. Poliwoda

Introduction

The prognosis for gastric carcinoma continues to be particularly unfavorable. Surgery can result in a cure or longer disease-free survival only in a small number of patients, since most gastric carcinomas are diagnosed when the tumor is in an advanced stage. More than 85% of all patients with newly diagnosed gastric carcinoma die from a nonresectable local tumor and/or distant metastases. For this reason, chemotherapy is the treatment of choice in cases of advanced gastric carcinoma, either alone or in combination with surgery and/or radiation therapy.

While objective response rates of 30% to 40% are achieved with the more frequently employed chemotherapy protocols such as FAM,[1-15] FAB,[16-20] and FAP,[21-28] complete remissions are rare (5%). A response rate of 73%, including 21% complete remissions, was achieved in 56 patients with advanced gastric carcinoma during a phase II study with the etoposide/Adriamycin/cisplatin (EAP) combination.[29] A comparison between EAP and other combinations (FAM, FAB, FAP) more frequently used in cases of gastric carcinoma indicates that EAP may be more effective. Complete remission was induced in 6 of 12 patients having only locally advanced gastric carcinoma. A radical resection of residual tumors was also shown to be possible after objective remissions induced by EAP.

EAP in Locally Advanced and Nonresectable Gastric Carcinoma

A disease-oriented phase II study in which EAP was employed as preoperative chemotherapy was therefore carried out in patients with locally advanced and nonresectable gastric carcinoma. A total of 27 patients with locally advanced and nonresectable gastric carcinoma were included in this study from June 1985 to July 1987. The most important criterion for inclusion was the execution of an exploratory laparotomy, during which tumor resectability and spread were determined. The definition of locally advanced gastric carcinoma was also expanded to include lymph-node participation in the N3 compartment (now M1 in abdominal lymph nodes according to the new UICC classification, in effect since

January 1, 1987) and local peritoneal carcinosis caused by tumor penetration into the serous membrane. The study design called for patients with locally advanced or nonresectable gastric carcinoma to receive chemotherapy with EAP following exploratory laparotomy. Chemotherapy was initiated 2 weeks after the operation in the case of exploratory laparotomy and 3 weeks postoperatively in the case of palliative surgery of the gastrointestinal tract. A second-look operation with resection of residual tumor was planned for patients in whom chemotherapy induced objective remissions (CR/PR). Both the exploratory laparotomy and second-look operation were performed by the same surgeon. Two additional EAP cycles were provided for consolidation in cases where the clinical remission was confirmed during the operation.

A remission rate of 70% was induced in 19 of the 27 patients, including 6 (22%) complete remissions. Two patients exhibited minor tumor responses or tumor stabilization (minor remission/no change), and the tumor was primarily progressive during chemotherapy in five patients. One patient died from a presumed tumor perforation (early death) 14 days into the initial chemotherapy. Sixteen of 19 patients showing an objective response to chemotherapy were subjected to a second-look operation. One patient with a clinically complete remission refused to undergo a second operation. Two patients with a clinically partial remission exhibited renewed tumor progression prior to the planned second-look operation. The clinically complete remission was confirmed pathologically in five patients. The tumor could be resected completely (RO) in eight cases (partial remissions). Tumor cells remained in the oral resection edge in two patients (Rl resection). Both patients were tumor-free for 5+ and 19+ months following consolidation therapy. The tumor became nonresectable again in one patient. A "down-staging" induced by the chemotherapy (comparison of the TNM stage determined during exploratory laparotomy against the TNM stage during the second-look operation) could be objectified in 14 of 15 tumors which became resectable following EAP (Table 1).

After a median observation time of 15 months, 5 of 16 patients were tumor-free after EAP ± surgery ± consolidation chemotherapy (1 cCr, 5 cPR, 10 NED), for a relapse rate of 33%. One patient died of brain metastasis, without further tumor localization found at autopsy. A female patient had a small local recurrence in the stomach. In her case, no tumor could be detected macroscopically during the second-look operation, and multiple biopsies from the previous tumor region also gave no indication of residual tumor. Gastrectomy was therefore not performed during the second-look operation. While the local relapse could be radically resected, the patient died from brain metastases as the sole tumor manifestation at autopsy. Two other patients had tumor recurrence in regional lymph nodes, and one patient had a local recurrence in the gastric layer. Other than these two CNS recurrences, distant metastases were not observed.

Median survival time for the overall group was 20.5 months (range 0.5–26+). The median disease-free interval and the median survival time for patients who were disease-free after EAP ± surgery ± consolidation chemotherapy with EAP is 25 months. No elevated peri- or postoperative morbidity rate was found in this

Table 1. Treatment results following EAP + second-look operation (n = 16)

Age	Stage b. Expl. Lap.	CR/PR	EAP Cycles (n)	Stage b. second-look	Surgical procedure[a]	Postoperative result
23	T4 N2 M0	cCR	4	pCR	G + L	pCR
61	Local recurrence + N3 M0	cCR	4 + 2	pCR	EL + MB	pCR
34	R2-resection + N3 M0	cCR	4 + 2	pCR	L + MB	pCR
18	T4 N3 M0	cCR	3 + 2	pCR	EL + MB	pCR
53	T4 N3 M0	cCR	4+ 2	pCR	G + L	pCR
64	T4 N3 M0	cPR	4 + 2	pT3 N3 M0	G + L	R1 resection[b]
63	T4 N1 M0	cPR	5 + 2	pT2 N1 M0	G + L	R1 resection[b]
54	T4 N3 M0	cPR	5	pT4 N3 M0	EL	Nonresectable
42	T4 N1 M0	cPR	4 + 2	pT1 N0 M0	G + L	NED
65	T4 N3 M0	cPR	4	pT3 N0 M0	G + L	NED
59	T4 N2 M0	cPR	3 + 1	pT3 N1 M0	G + L	NED
65	T4 N2 M0	cPR	2	pT4 N2 M0	G + L	NED
57	T4 N3 M0	cPR	6 + 1	pT2 N3 M0	G + L	NED
55	T4 N2 M0	cPR	3 + 1	pT2 N1 M0	G + L	NED
59	T3 N1 M0	cPR	4 + 2	pT2 N1 M0	G + L	NED
57	T4 N3 M0	cPR	4 + 1	pT2 N0 M0	G + L	NED

[a] G = gastrectomy, L = lymphadenectomy, EL = exploratory laparotomy, MB = multiple biopsies.
[b] Without indication for tumor after two consolidation cycles with EAP.

study in patients treated with chemotherapy prior to the operation in comparison to surgery alone without neoadjuvant, perioperative, or postadjuvant chemotherapy. No deaths caused by chemotherapy or surgery were observed.

Discussion

Experience with preoperative chemotherapy in patients with locally advanced gastric carcinoma is limited. Only a handful of clinical studies,[30–33] and a few more case reports[34,35] address this mode of therapy. Stephens and associates[32] reported that 11 of 27 patients remained free of disease between 1 and 5 years following surgery when FAM and BCNU were administered intraarterially prior to the operation. No differences in survival time between patients receiving neoadjuvant treatment and historical control groups could be found in two other nonrandomized studies.[30,31] The only published randomized study involved the intravenous administration of mitomycin and showed that patients treated prior to the operation in stage III had an advantage in terms of survival time.[33]

In a small study with preoperatively administered FAM, five objective remissions were induced in five patients with locally advanced and clinically nonresectable gastric carcinoma.[35] Three resections could be carried out, with residual tumor detected in the resected stomach in all three cases (one microscopically and two macroscopically).

Surgically confirmed nonresectability of the primary tumor was not an essential criterion for inclusion in any of these studies. It is therefore not possible to arrive at a conclusion as to whether the preoperative chemotherapy contributed to the resectability and survival or whether surgery alone could have yielded the same results. The relatively slight effectiveness of the more frequently employed treatment protocols such as FAM and FAM modifications (response rate 30% to 35%; median duration of remission 5 to 9 months; median survival time 7 months) might explain why only a handful of studies have focused on the effectiveness of preoperative chemotherapy in gastric carcinoma. It could nonetheless be shown in other tumor entities that chemotherapy which is not all that effective in advanced tumors can be very effective in lower tumor stages, especially in combination with surgery and/or radiation therapy.[36–38]

The following considerations and experimental results make up the theoretical foundation for the concept behind preoperative chemotherapy.

- The probability of primary, frequently pleiotropically resistant cell populations grows as the size of the tumor increases. One would therefore expect chemotherapy to be more effective at a lower tumor mass (early tumor stages).[39,40] Animals with transplanted xenograft tumors clearly lived longer when chemotherapy was administered preoperatively rather than postoperatively.[41,42]
- The regional vascular supply is changed considerably following tumor resection. This could lead to the reduced exposure of the residual tumor in the area of the operation to cytostatic agents.[43,44]

The theoretical experimental foundations and promising clinical results obtained with preoperative chemotherapy in other tumors (eg, osteosarcoma, tumors of the head and neck[36,37]) were the basis for this study.

The etoposide/ADM/CDDP combination was selected for its high level of effectiveness in patients with highly advanced gastric carcinoma. The objective of this study was to enable radical resection in patients with primary nonresectable gastric carcinoma by a chemotherapeutically induced reduction of the locoregional tumor. Effectiveness of EAP on occult distant metastases was also to be assessed. Another important goal was concerned with checking the feasibility of a second-look operation following preoperative chemotherapy.

This study confirms the effectiveness of EAP in advanced gastric carcinoma.[29] The goal of enabling secondary resectability following preoperative chemotherapy was reached in a high percentage—56% (15 of 27)—of patients. Five complete and ten partial remissions could be surgically and pathologically confirmed.

Compared with image-generating procedures such as CT, sonography, and endoscopy, the second-look operation is much more precise in terms of assessing the remission. This procedure helps to identify subgroups of patients who might benefit from postoperative chemotherapy. In addition, the resected tumor material may be used for testing the sensitivity of chemotherapy.

In excess of 60% of all patients with resected, locally advanced gastric carcinoma normally develop distant metastases, whether alone or in combination with local relapses.[45] Apart from the two recurrent CNS metastases, which represent the exception in cases of gastric carcinoma, no other distant metastases were found in this study. As an agent for preoperative chemotherapy, therefore, EAP appears to be highly effective at destroying distant metastases. The four regional relapses observed previously (one in the stomach, two in the lymph nodes, one in the stomach layer) suggest that the resection performed during the second-look operation should be as radical as possible (gastrectomy, expanded lymphadenectomy). The median life expectancy for untreated patients with locally advanced and nonresectable gastric carcinoma is about 4 months.[46,47] When treated with standard chemotherapy protocols (FAM; FAM modifications), their survival time is approximately 7 months.* The median survival time measured 21 months in this study, 25 months for patients with NED after EAP $\pm$ surgery $\pm$ consolidation chemotherapy.

EAP as an agent for preoperative chemotherapy seems to improve the prognosis for patients with locally advanced gastric carcinoma and may help heal some of these patients for whom the prognosis would otherwise be fatal. In light of these promising results, the concept of preoperative chemotherapy in cases of gastric carcinoma should be examined in other well-planned studies.

References

1. Beretta G, Fraschini P, Labianca R, et al: The value of FAM polychemotherapy in advanced gastric carcinoma, abstract C-400. Proc ASCO 1982;1:103.
2. Beretta G, Fraschini P, Labianca R, et al: Weekly 5-fluorouracil (F) versus combination chemotherapy for advanced gastrointestinal carcinomas. A prospective study program, abstract C-367. Proc ASCO 1986;5:94.
3. Biran H, Sulkes A: A possible dose-response relationship in "FAM" chemotherapy for advanced gastric cancer, abstract C-515. Proc ASCO 1984;3:132.
4. Cartei G: 5-Fluorouracil, Adriamycin und Mitomycin C beim Magenkarzinom, in Nagel GA, Bach F, Bartsch HH (eds): Aktuelle Onkologie. Munich-Bern-Vienna, W. Zuckschwerdt, 1985, p 56.
5. Douglass HO Jr, Lavin PT, Goudsmit A, et al: An Eastern Cooperative Oncology Group evaluation of combinations of methyl-CCNU, mitomycin C, Adriamycin, and 5-fluorouracil in advanced measurable gastric cancer (EST 2277). J Clin Oncol 1984;2:1372.
6. Fornasiero A, Cartei G, Daniele O, et al: FAM2 regimen in disseminated gastric cancer. Tumori 1984;70:77.
7. Haas C, Oishi N, McDonald B, et al: Southwest Oncology Group phase II-III gastric cancer study: 5-fluorouracil, Adriamycin, and mitomycin C + vincristine (FAM vs V-FAM) compared to chlorozotocin (CZT), M-AMSA, and dihydroxyanthracenedione (DHAD) with unimpressive differences, abstract C-478. Proc ASCO 1983;2:122.
8. Haim N, Cohen Y, Honigman J, et al: Treatment of advanced gastric carcinoma with 5-fluorouracil, Adriamycin, and mitomycin C (FAM). Cancer Chemother Pharmacol 1982;8:277.

*Refs. 1,2,3,4,5,6,7,8,9,10,11,12,13,14,15.

9. Haim N, Epelbaum R, Cohen Y, et al: Further studies in the treatment of advanced gastric cancer by 5-fluorouracil, Adriamycin (doxorubicin), and mitomycin C (modified FAM). Cancer 1984;54:1999.
10. Kim NK: Chemotherapy of advanced gastric carcinoma with 5-fluorouracil, Adriamycin, mitomycin (FAM), and 5-fluorouracil, Adriamycin, cisplatin (FAP) combinations: experience in Korea, in Ogawa M, Muggia FM, Rozencweig M (eds): Adriamycin, Its Expanding Role in Cancer Treatment. Amsterdam, Excerpta Medica, 1984, p 137.
11. MacDonald JS, Schein PS, Woolley PV, et al: 5-Fluorouracil, doxorubicin, and mitomycin (FAM) combination-chemotherapy for advanced gastric cancer. Ann Intern Med 1980;93:533.
12. Oshima K, Yamada T, Nonaka T, et al: Treatment of advanced GI cancer with 5-FU, Adriamycin, and mitomycin C (FAM). Proc 13th Intern Cancer Congr Seattle, 1982, abstract 695.
13. Pannettiere FJ, Haas C, McDonald B, et al: Drug combinations in the treatment of gastric adenocarcinoma: a randomized Southwest Oncology Group study. J Clin Oncol 1984;2:420.
14. The Gastrointestinal Tumor Study Group: Phase II-III chemotherapy studies in advanced gastric cancer. Cancer Treat Rep 1979;63:1871.
15. The Gastrointestinal Tumor Study Group: Randomized study of combination chemotherapy in unresectable gastric cancer. Cancer 1984;53:13.
16. Levi JA, Dalley DN, Aroney RS: Improved combination chemotherapy in advanced gastric cancer. Br Med J 1979;2:1471.
17. Levi JA, Fox RM, Tattersall MH, et al: Analysis of a prospective randomized comparison of doxorubicin versus 5-fluorouracil, doxorubicin, and BCNU in advanced gastric cancer: implications for future studies. J Clin Oncol 1986;4:1348.
18. Lopez M, Di Lauro L, Papaldo P, et al: Treatment of advanced measurable gastric carcinoma with 5-fluorouracil, Adriamycin, and BCNU. Oncology 1986;43:288.
19. Lopez M, Perno CF, Di Lauro L, Papaldo P: 5-Fluorouracil, Adriamycin, BCNU (FAB) combination chemotherapy for advanced gastric cancer. Cancer Chemother Pharmacol 1984;12:194.
20. Schnitzler G, Queisser W, Heim ME, et al: Phase III study of 5-FU and carmustine versus 5-FU, carmustine, and doxorubicin in advanced gastric cancer. Cancer Treat Rep 1986;70:477.
21. Cazap EL, Gisselbrecht C, Smith FP, et al: Phase II trials of 5-FU, doxorubicin, and cisplatin in advanced, measurable adenocarcinoma of the lung and stomach. Cancer Treat Rep 1986;70:781.
22. Figoli F, Galligioni E, Crivellari D, et al: Cisplatin (DDP) in combination with Adriamycin (A) and fluorouracil (F) (DAF) in advanced gastric cancer—a phase II study, abstract C-369. Proc ASCO 1986;5:95.
23. Moertel CG, Fleming T, O'Connell MJ, et al: A phase II study of combined 5-fluorouracil, doxorubicin, and cisplatin in the treatment of advanced upper gastrointestinal adenocarcinomas. J Clin Oncol 1986;4:1053.
24. Moertel CG, Rubin J, O'Connell MJ, et al: A phase II study of combined 5-fluorouracil, doxorubicin, and cisplatin in the treatment of advanced upper gastrointestinal adenocarcinomas. J Clin Oncol 1986;4:1053.
25. Robinson E, Haim N, Epelbaum R, et al: Phase II trials in the treatment of advanced gastric cancer, I—5-fluorouracil, Adriamycin and mitomycin (FAM), II—cisplatin, Adriamycin and 5-fluorouracil (DAF), abstract C-300. Proc ASCO 1985;4:77.

26. Rougier P, Droz JP, Amiel JL, et al: Gastric carcinoma: a phase II trial of chemotherapy with association 5-fluorouracil (5 FU), Adriamycin (ADR) and cisplatin (DDP) (FAP protocol) in metastasized or inoperable patients. Preliminary results. Cancer Chemother Pharmacol 1985;14(suppl):54.
27. Wagener DJT, Yap SH, Wobbes T, et al: Phase II trial of 5-fluorouracil, Adriamycin, and cisplatin (FAP) in advanced gastric cancer. Cancer Chemother Pharmacol 1985;15:86.
28. Woolley P, Smith F, Estevez R, et al: A phase II trial of 5-FU, Adriamycin and cisplatin (FAP) in advanced gastric cancer, abstract C-481. Proc ASCO 1981;455.
29. Preusser P, Wilke H, Achterrath W, et al: Advanced gastric carcinoma: a phase II study with etoposide (E), Adriamycin (A) and split course cisplatin (P) = EAP. Proc ASCO 1987;6:292.
30. Fujimoto S, Akao T, Itol B, et al: A study of survival in patients with stomach cancer treated by a combination of preoperative intra-arterial infusion therapy and surgery. Cancer 1976;37:1648.
31. Nishioka B, Ouchi T, Watanabe S, et al: Follow-up study of preoperative oral administration of an antineoplastic agent as an adjuvant chemotherapy in gastric cancer. Gan To Kagaku Ryoho 1982;9:1427.
32. Stephens FO, Johnson AW, Crea P: Preoperative "basal" chemotherapy in the management of cancer of the stomach. Med J Aust 1984;140:143.
33. Jinnai D, Higashi H: Extended radical operation with preoperative chemotherapy for gastric cancer, in Hirayama T (ed): Cancer in Asia. Baltimore, University Park Press, 1976, p 111.
34. Klein HO: Preoperative chemotherapy in patients with gastric cancer. Prog Clin Biol Res 1985;201:283.
35. Bonatsos C, Aust J, Meisner D, et al: Preoperative chemotherapy for patients with locally advanced gastric cancer (abstract). Proc ASCO 1985;4:83.
36. Clark JR, Fallon BG, Frei III E: Induction chemotherapy as initial treatment for advanced head and neck cancer: a model for the multidisciplinary treatment of solid tumors, in DeVita VT, Hellman S, Rosenberg SA (eds): Important Advances in Oncology. Philadelphia, Lippincott, 1987, p 175.
37. Rosen G, Nirenberg A: Neoadjuvant chemotherapy for osteogenic sarcoma: a five-year follow-up (T-10) and preliminary report of new studies (T-12), in Wagener DJT, Blijham GH, Smeets JBE, et al (eds): Primary Chemotherapy in Cancer Medicine. New York, Alan R. Liss, 1985, p 39.
38. Advani SJ, Saiki TK, Swaroop S, et al: Anterior chemotherapy in esophageal cancer. Cancer 1985;56:1502.
39. Goldie JH, Coldman AJ: A mathematical model for relating the sensitivity of tumors to their spontaneous mutation rate. Cancer Treat Rep 1979;63:1727.
40. Goldie JH, Coldman AJ: Quantitative model for multiple levels of drug resistance in clinical tumors. Cancer Treat Rep 1983;67:923.
41. Fisher D, Gunduz N, Saffer EA: Influence of the interval between primary tumor removal and chemotherapy on kinetics and growth of metastases. Cancer Res 1983;43:1488.
42. Van Putten LM: Optimal timing of adjuvant chemotherapy in mouse models, in Wagener DJT, Blijham GH, Smeets JBE, et al (eds): Primary Chemotherapy in Cancer Medicine. New York, Alan R. Liss, 1985, p 15.
43. Rubin P, Casarett GW: Clinical Radiation Pathology. Philadelphia, WB Saunders, 1968.

44. Reinhold HS, Buisman GH: Radiosensitivity of capillary endothelium. Br J Radiol 1973;46:54.
45. Meyer HJ, Pichmayr R: Patterns of recurrence to therapeutic strategy in gastric cancer. Scand J Gastroenterol 1986;22:45.
46. Trompke R, Grege A, Keser M: Zum natürlichen Verlauf des Magenkrebses. Bruns' Beitr Klin Chir 1965;211:19.
47. Moertel CG: The natural history of advanced gastric cancer. Surg Gynec Obstet 1968;126:1071.

CHAPTER 15

Chemotherapy of Advanced Gastric Carcinoma in Elderly and High-Risk Patients

P. Preusser, H. Wilke, W. Achterrath, and U. Fink

Introduction

Gastric carcinoma is the second leading cause of death in cases of malignant neoplasias in the Federal Republic of Germany. A total of 28 of 100,000 inhabitants die from gastric carcinoma every year.[1]

Approximately 60% of patients with gastric carcinoma are older than 65 years of age.[2] Only about 20% of the patients are treated within studies for reasons of advanced age and/or comorbidity.[3] These facts necessitate the development of chemotherapy programs for elderly patients (older than 65 years of age).

Only a few effective cytostatic drugs are currently available for the chemotherapeutic treatment of gastric carcinoma based upon a remission rate of greater than 15% as the activity limit.[4]

Numerous cytostatic agents have been tested in disease-oriented phase II studies involving patients without prior chemotherapy since 1980. Idarubicin,[5] aclacinomycin,[6] mitoxantrone,[6,7] bisanthrene,[6] amsacrine,[8] and roxazone[6] had little or no effect (remission rate <10%).

Table 1 shows substances identified as effective in disease-oriented phase II studies with more than 14 patients. Etoposide showed activity comparable to the other substances listed, although dosage was only 30% to 50% of the dosage recommended for phase II studies.[9-12]

The cytostatic agents identified as effective were tested in numerous combinations during the course of open and disease-oriented studies, with combinations of three cytostatic drugs primarily being employed more recently. Table 2 summarizes the therapeutic results. Analysis of the studies shows that 27% to 43% remissions (2% to 11% complete remissions) were achieved with the more frequently used combinations FAM, FAB, FAMe, FAMTX, and FAP. Median duration of remission was 5 to 9 months in the majority of studies, while the median survival time for all patients was 6 to 8 months.

A complete remission rate of 22% and an overall remission rate of 71% were achieved in 72 patients during a disease-oriented phase I/II study with the EAP combination. These data indicate that within the 95% confidence limits EAP induces higher remission rates than the other combinations. Median duration of

Table 1. Monoactivity in patients with gastric carcinoma not pretreated with chemotherapy (remission rate >15%)

Substance	No. of patients	CR n	CR %	CR + PR n	CR + PR %	mR	Reference
5-FU	54	1	2	11	20	4	a,b,c,d
ADM	124	10	8	21	17	4–6	d,e,f,g
Epi-ADM	39	2	5	8	21	NS	h
CDDP	14	2	14	5	36	3–6	i
Etoposide	14		0	3	21	1^{+}–5	j
Mitomycin C	211		NS	63	30	NS	k,l
BCNU	55	1	2	10	18	5	d,m

NS = not stated.

[a] Cocconi G, De Lisi V, Di Blasio B: Randomized comparison of 5-FU alone or combined with mitomycin and cytarabine (MFC) in the treatment of advanced gastric cancer. Cancer Treat Rep 1982;66:1263.

[b] De Lisi V, Cocconi G, Tonato M, et al: Randomized comparison of 5-FU alone or combined with carmustine, and mitomycin (BAFMi) in the treatment of advanced gastric cancer: a phase III trial of the Italian Clinical Research Oncology Group (GOIRC). Cancer Treat Rep 1986;70:481.

[c] Kolaric K, Potrebica V, Stanovnik M: Controlled phase III clinical study of 4 epi-doxorubicin + 5-fluorouracil versus 5-fluorouracil alone in metastatic gastric and rectosigmoid cancer. Oncology 1986;43:73.

[d] MacDonald JS, Gunderson LL, Cohn I Jr: Cancer of the stomach, in DeVita VT, Hellman S, Rosenberg SA (eds): Cancer: Principles and Practices of Oncology. Philadelphia, Lippincott, 1985, p 534.

[e] Levi JA, Fox RM, Tattersall MH, et al: Analysis of a prospective randomized comparison of doxorubicin versus 5-fluorouracil, doxorubicin, and BCNU in advanced gastric cancer: implications for future studies. J Clin Oncol 1986;4:1348.

[f] Moertel CG, Lavin PT: Phase II–III chemotherapy studies in advanced gastric cancer. Cancer Treat Rep 1979;63:1863.

[g] The Gastrointestinal Tumor Study Group: Phase II–III chemotherapy studies in advanced gastric cancer. Cancer Treat Rep 1979;63:1871.

[h] Walder S, Green M, Muggia F: The role of anthracyclines in the treatment of gastric cancer. Cancer Treat Rev 1985;12:105.

[i] Leichmann L, MacDonald B, Dindogru A, et al: Platinum: a clinical active drug in advanced adenocarcinoma of the stomach, abstract. Proc Am Asso Cancer Res 1982;110:430.

[j] Kelsen DP, Magill C, Cheng E, et al: Phase II trial of etoposide (VP16) in the treatment of upper gastrointestinal malignancies, abstract. Proc ASCO 1982;96:C-371.

[k] Comis RL: Mitomycin C in gastric cancer, in Carter SK, Crooke ST (eds): Mitomycin C–Current Status and New Developments. New York, Academic Press, 1979, p 129.

[l] Schein PS, MacDonald JS, Hoth D, et al: Mitomycin C: experience in the United States, with emphasis on gastric cancer. Cancer Chemother Pharmacol 1978;1:73.

[m] Moertel CG: Therapy of advanced gastrointestinal cancer with the nitrosoureas. Cancer Chemother Rep 1973;4:27.

Table 2. Summary of results with the more frequently used combinations of 3 cytostatic agents (>50 patients)

Combination	No. of patients	No. of studies	CR n	CR %	CR + PR n	CR + PR %	mR (mon)	mS (mon)	Reference
FAM	612	14	10	2	185	30	5–10	6–9⁺	a,b,c,d,e,f,g,h,i,j, k,l,m,n,o
					26%–34%*				
FAMe	55	2	6	11	15	27	5	6	e,o
					15%–39%*				
FAB	177	4	10	6	76	43	7–9	6–8	p,q,r,s,t
					36%–50%*				
FAP	187	8	9	5	68	36	4,5–7	6–13	j,u,v,w,x,y,z,aa, bb
					29%–43%*				
FAMTX	187	3	21	11	81	43	9	3–8	cc,dd,ee
					36%–50%				
EAP	72	2	16	22	51	71	7	9	ff,gg
					60%–82%*				

*95% confidence limits.

[a] Beretta G, Fraschini P, Labianca R, et al: The value of FAM polychemotherapy in advanced gastric carcinoma, abstract. Proc ASCO 1982;103:C-400.

[b] Beretta G, Fraschini P, Labianca R, et al: Weekly 5-fluorouracil (F) versus combination chemotherapy for advanced gastrointestinal carcinomas. A prospective study program, abstract. Proc ASCO 1986;94:C-367.

[c] Biran H, Sulkes A: A possible dose-response relationship in "FAM" chemotherapy for advanced gastric cancer, abstract. Proc ASCO 1984;132:C-515.

[d] Cartei G: 5-Fluorouracil, Adriamycin und Mitomycin C beim metastasierenden Magenkarzinom, in Nagel GA, Bach F, Bartsch HH (eds): Mitomycin '85, Aktuelle Onkologie, Munich, W. Zuckerschwerdt, 1985, p 56.

[e] Douglass HO Jr, Lavin PT, Goudsmit A, et al: An Eastern Cooperative Oncology Group evaluation of combinations of methyl-CCNU, mitomycin C, Adriamycin, and 5-fluorouracil in advanced measurable gastric cancer (EST 2277). J Clin Oncol 1984;2:1372.

[f] Fornasiero A, Cartei G, Daniele O, et al: FAM2 regimen in disseminated gastric cancer. Tumori 1984;70:77.

[g] Haas C, Oishi N, McDonald B, et al: Southwest Oncology Group phase II–III gastric cancer study: 5-fluorouracil, Adriamycin, and mitomycin C + vincristine (FAM vs V-FAM) compared to Chlorozotocin (CZT), M-AMSA, and Dihydroxyanthracenedione (DHAD) with unimpressive differences, abstract. Proc ASCO 1983;122:C-478.

[h] Haim N, Cohen Y, Honigman J, et al: Treatment of advanced gastric carcinoma with 5-fluorouracil, Adriamycin, and mitomycin C (FAM): Cancer Chemother Pharmacol 1982;8:277.

[i] Haim N, Epelbaum R, Cohen Y, et al: Further studies in the treatment of advanced gastric cancer by 5-fluorouracil, Adriamycin (doxorubicin), and Mitomycin C (modified FAM). Cancer 1984;54: 1999.

[j] Kim NK: Chemotherapy of advanced gastric carcinoma with 5-fluorouracil, Adriamycin, mitomycin (FAM), and 5-fluorouracil, Adriamycin, cisplatin (FAP) combinations: experience in Korea, in Ogawa M, Muggia FM, Rozencweig M (eds): Adriamycin, Its Expanding Role in Cancer Treatment. Amsterdam, Excerpta Medica, 1984, p 137.

[k] MacDonald JS, Schein PS, Woolley PV, et al: 5-Fluorouracil, doxorubicin, and mitomycin (FAM) combination-chemotherapy for advanced gastric cancer. Ann Intern Med 1980;93:533.

[l] Oshima K, Yamada T, Nonaka T, et al: Treatment of advanced G.I. cancer patients with 5-FU, Adriamycin, and mitomycin C (FAM). Abstract 3977, Proc 13th Inter Cancer Congress, Seattle 8–15 Sept 1982, p 665.

Table 2. *Continued.*

[m]Pannettiere FJ, Haas C, McDonald B, et al: Drug combinations in the treatment of gastric adenocarcinoma: a randomized Southwest Oncology Group study. J Clin Oncol 1984;2:420.
[n]The Gastrointestinal Tumor Study Group: Phase II–III chemotherapy studies in advanced gastric cancer. Cancer Treat Rep 1979;63:1871.
[o]The Gastrointestinal Tumor Study Group: Randomized study of combination chemotherapy in unresectable gastric cancer. Cancer 1984;53:13.
[p]Levi JA, Dalley DN, Aroney RS: Improved combination chemotherapy in advanced gastric cancer. Br Med J 1979;2:1471.
[q]Levi JA, Fox RM, Tattersall MH, et al: Analysis of a prospective randomized comparison of doxorubicin versus 5-fluorouracil, doxorubicin, and BCNU in advanced gastric cancer: implications for future studies. J Clin Oncol 1986;4:1348.
[r]Lopez M, Di Lauro L, Papaldo P, et al: Treatment of advanced measurable gastric carcinoma with 5-fluorouracil, Adriamycin, and BCNU. Oncology 1986;43:288.
[s]Lopez M, Perno CF, Di Lauro L, et al: 5-Fluorouracil, Adriamycin, BCNU (FAB) combination chemotherapy for advanced gastric cancer. Cancer Chemother Pharmacol 1984;12:194.
[t]Schnitzler G, Queisser W, Heim ME, et al: Phase III study of 5-FU and carmustine versus 5-FU, carmustine, and doxorubicin in advanced gastric cancer. Cancer Treat Rep 1986;70:477.
[u]Cazap EL, Gisselbrecht C, Smith FP, et al: Phase II trials of 5-FU, doxorubicin, and cisplatin in advanced, measurable adenocarcinoma of the lung and stomach. Cancer Treat Rep 1986;70:781.
[v]Figoli F, Galligioni E, Crivellari D, et al: Cisplatin (DDP) in combination with Adriamycin (A) and fluorouracil (F) (DAF) in advanced gastric cancer—a phase II study, abstract. Proc ASCO 1986;95:C-369.
[w]Moertel CG, Fleming T, O'Connell M, et al: A phase II trial of combined intensive course 5-FU, Adriamycin and cis-platinum in advanced gastric and pancreatic carcinoma, abstract. Proc ASCO 1984;137:C-535.
[x]Moertel CG, Rubin J, O'Connell MJ, et al: A phase II study of combined 5-fluorouracil, doxorubicin, and cisplatin in the treatment of advanced upper gastrointestinal adenocarcinomas. J Clin Oncol 1986;4:1053.
[y]Robinson E, Haim N, Epelbaum R, et al: Phase II trials in the treatment of advanced gastric cancer I—5-fluorouracil, Adriamycin and mitomycin (FAM), II—cisplatin, Adriamycin and 5-fluorouracil (DAF), abstract. Proc ASCO 1985;77:C-300.
[z]Rougier P, Droz JP, Amiel JL, et al: Gastric carcinoma: a phase II trial of chemotherapy with association 5-fluorouracil (5 FU), Adriamycin (ADR) and cisplatin (DDP) (FAP protocol) in metastasized or inoperable patients. Preliminary results. Cancer Chemother Pharmacol 1985;14(suppl):54.
[aa]Wagener DJT, Yap SH, Wobbes T, et al: Phase II trial of 5-fluorouracil, Adriamycin, and cisplatin (FAP) in advanced gastric cancer. Cancer Chemother Pharmacol 1985;15:86.
[bb]Woolley P, Smith F, Estevez R, et al: A phase II trial of 5-FU, Adriamycin and cisplatin (FAP) in advanced gastric cancer, abstract. Proc ASCO 1981;455:C-481.
[cc]Herrmann R, Fritze D, Queisser W, et al: Chemotherapie des Magenkarzinoms. Dtsch Med Wochenschr 1984;109:1704.
[dd]Klein HO, Wickramanyake PD, Farkh GR: 5-fluorouracil (5-FU), Adriamycin (ADM), and methotrexate (MTX)—a combination protocol (FAMTX) for treatment of metastasized stomach cancer, abstract. Proc ASCO 1986;84:C-325.
[ee]Wils J, Bleiberg H, Dalesio O, et al: An EORTC gastrointestinal group evaluation of the combination of sequential methotrexate and 5-fluorouracil, combined with Adriamycin in advanced measurable gastric cancer. J Clin Oncol 1987;4:1799.
[ff]Preusser P, Wilke H, Achterrath W, et al: Advanced inoperable stomach cancer: a pilot study with the combination etoposide, Adriamycin, and cisplatin. Anticancer Res 1986;6:1195.
[gg]Preusser P, Wilke H, Achterrath W, et al: Advanced gastric carcinoma: a phase II study with etoposide (E), Adriamycin (A), and split course cisplatin (P) = EAP, abstract. Proc ASCO 1987;6:292.

remission and survival time of patients treated with EAP rank in the upper third of published data.

Most cytostatic agents used more frequently in the chemotherapy of gastric carcinoma show syntropic and/or cumulative organ toxicity, as a result of which unexpected and/or serious side effects may be induced (Table 3). Of considerable therapeutic importance is the delayed onset and long duration of the myelosuppressive effect induced by BCNU and mitomycin C, which increase the danger of infection and hemorrhage. The cumulative effect which both substances have on the bone marrow and lungs may necessitate early reductions in dose and can induce fatal complications.

ADM and epi-ADM may only be employed on a restricted basis in patients with heart disease in light of their potential cardiotoxicity. The cardiotoxic effect exhibited by both substances is cumulative and limits the overall administrable dose.* A reduction in the cumulative dose of doxorubicin would seem justified with respect to single-drug therapy in light of the possibly additive cardiotoxicity of ADM and mitomycin C.[13]

Because of its spectrum of side effects, CDDP is an important constituent in the polychemotherapy of gastric carcinoma. Myelosuppression induced by CDDP is not pronounced at usual doses (≤ 100 mg/m^2). In contrast, myelosuppression represents the acute dose-limiting side effect for the other effective cytostatic drugs. Clear reductions in dosages of the constituents in a combination are therefore necessary in polychemotherapy as opposed to single-drug therapy when only cytostatic drugs with a pronounced myelosuppressive effect are used.

Dosage reductions may to a large extent be avoided in the other effective substances by replacing cytostatic agents which exert a myelosuppressive effect at normal dosages with CDDP. Therapy with CDDP is frequently complicated by nausea and vomiting as well as complicated hydration programs for preventing disturbances of renal function. In addition, polyneuropathies and ototoxicity limit the duration of treatment. The frequency and severity of these two side effects correlate primarily with the cumulatively administered dose of CDDP.

5-FU and etoposide apparently have no serious and/or cumulative organ toxicity. Their myelosuppressive effect depends on the dose, may be reversed in relatively short order, and can be predicted with accuracy. General tolerance to both substances is relatively good.

The range of side effects associated with the cytostatic agents currently used mostly in combinations shows that chemotherapeutic regimens such as FAM, FAMe, FAP, FAB, FAMTX, and EAP should only be administered within studies on strictly selected groups of patients. Only patients up to 65 years of age with sufficient bone marrow, heart, liver, and kidney function are as a rule included in clinical studies. Since only about 20% of all patients satisfy these strict selection criteria, 80% must be treated outside of studies.[3] The situation is similar in patients with advanced gastric carcinoma; as many as 60% of the patients are

*Myelosuppression is the acute dose-limiting toxicity.

Table 3. Serious side effects of cytostatic agents active against gastric carcinoma

Substance	Myelosuppression*	Other serious organ toxicity	Cumulative organ toxicity (references)
ADM	Acute dose-limiting; early, rapid recovery	Heart; cumulative dose-limiting	Heart (a,b)
Epi-ADM	Acute dose-limiting; early, rapid recovery	Heart, cumulative dose-limiting	Heart (c,d)
Mitomycin C	Acute dose-limiting, delayed onset, slow recovery	Lungs, kidney	Bone marrow, lungs (e)
BCNU	Acute dose-limiting, delayed onset, slow recovery	Lungs, kidney	Bone marrow, lungs (f,g)
CDDP	Not very pronounced at normal dosage	Peripheral nervous system, hearing GI tract	Peripheral nervous system, hearing, kidney? (h-t)
5-FU	Acute dose-limiting, early, rapid recovery	Mucositis, GI tract	(u)
Etoposide	Acute dose-limiting, early, rapid recovery	–	(b,v,w)

*Onset: early, nadir no later than day 16; delayed; nadir after > 3 weeks.
Recovery: rapid, within 20 days; slow, > 5 weeks.

[a] Dorr RT, Fritz WL: Doxorubicin, in Cancer Chemotherapy Handbook. New York, Elsevier, 1980, p 388.

[b] Radice PA, Bunn PA, Ihde DC: Therapeutic trials with VP-16-213 and VM-26: active agents in small cell lung cancer, non-Hodgkin's lymphomas, and other malignancies. Cancer Treat Rep 1977;63:1231.

[c] Ceresosismo RJ, Hong WK: Epirubicin: a review of pharmacology, clinical activity, and adverse effects of an Adriamycin analogue. J Clin Oncol 1986;4:425.

[d] Weiss RB, Sarosy G, Clagett-Carr K, et al: Anthracycline analogs: the past, present, and future. Cancer Chemother Pharmacol 1986;18:185.

[e] Doll DC, Weiss RB, Issell BF: Mitomycin: ten years after approval for marketing. J Clin Oncol 1985;3:276.

[f] Dorr RT, Fritz WL: Carmustine, in Cancer Chemotherapy Handbook. New York, Elsevier, 1980, p 295.

[g] Hunter CP, Frelick RW, Feldman AR, et al: Selection factors in clinical trials: results from the community clinical oncology program physician's patient log. Cancer Treat Rep 1987;71:559.

[h] Achterrath W, Raettig R, Franks CR, et al: Aktuelle Cisplatinderivate. Beitr Onkol 1984;18:58.

[i] Bonomi PB, Blessing JA, Stehmann FB, et al: Randomized trial of three cisplatin dose schedules in squamous-cell carcinoma of the cervix: a gynecologic oncology group study. J Clin Oncol 1985;3:1079.

[j] Fausti SA, Schechter MA, Rappaport BZ, et al: Early detection of cisplatin ototoxicity. Cancer 1984;53:224.

[k] Kris MG, Gralla RJ, Clark RA, et al: Incidence, course, and severity of delayed nausea and vomiting following the administration of high-dose cisplatin. J Clin Oncol 1985;3:1379.

[l] Legha SS, Dimery IW: High-dose cisplatin administration without hypertonic saline: observation of disabling neurotoxicity. J Clin Oncol 1985;3:1373.

[m] Melamed LB, Selim MA, Schuchman D: Cisplatin ototoxicity in gynecologic cancer patients. Cancer 1985;55:41.

[n] Ozols RF, Ostchega Y, Meyers CE, et al: High-dose cisplatin in hypertonic saline in refractory ovarian carcinoma. J Clin Oncol 1985;3:1246.

Table 3. *Continued.*

[o] Preusser P, Achterrath W, Niederle N, et al: Cisplatin. Arzneimitteltherapie 1985;2:50.
[p] Roelofs RI, Hrushesky W, Rogin J, et al: Peripheral sensory neuropathy and cisplatin chemotherapy. Neurology 1984;34:934.
[q] Schaefer SD, Post JD, Close LG, et al: Ototoxicity of low- and moderate-dose cisplatin. Cancer 1985;56:1934.
[r] Vermorken JB, Kapteijn TS, Hart AAM, et al: Ototoxicity of cis-diamminedichloroplatinum (II): influence of dose, schedule, and mode of administration. J Cancer Clin Oncol 1983;19:55.
[s] Wiltshaw E: Chemotherapy of ovarian malignancies at the Royal Marsden Hospital, in Bender HG, Beck L (eds): Carcinoma of the Ovary. Stuttgart, Fischer, 1983, p 169.
[t] Wiltshaw E, Evans B, Rustin G, et al: A prospective randomized trial comparing high-dose cisplatin with low-dose cisplatin and chlorambucil in advanced ovarian carcinoma. J Clin Oncol 1986;4:722.
[u] Dorr RT, Fritz WL: 5-Fluorouracil, in Cancer Chemotherapy Handbook. New York, Elsevier, 1980, p 435.
[v] O'Dwyer PJ, Leyland-Jones B, Alonso MT, et al: Etoposide (VP-16 213). N Engl J Med 1985;312:692.
[w] Schmoll HJ, Niederle N, Achterrath W: Etoposide (VP-16-213). Klin Wochenschr 1981;59:1177.

older than 65 years.[2] As is typical for this age group, they suffer from one or several organ diseases not caused by tumors, with the heart, kidneys, lungs and liver standing at the forefront.[14–16] Elevated sensitivity of the bone marrow and nervous system is likely in this age group as well.[17]

The age-dependent comorbidity rates and elevated organ sensitivity (especially of the bone marrow) make it necessary to develop special risk-adapted chemotherapy programs for elderly patients (older than 65 years of age and high-risk patients). Effective cytostatic drugs which have good overall tolerance, accurately predictable side effects and slight, non-cumulative organ toxicity should be employed primarily in the development of these programs, since palliation is still the focus of all therapeutic efforts.

Of the cytostatic agents effective against gastric carcinoma, 5-FU and etoposide satisfy these requirements the best. Phase II studies published by several groups indicate that the effectiveness of 5-FU in treating gastric carcinoma may be enhanced by the simultaneous administration of LV.[18,19] The clinical data presented indicate that the LV/5-FU/etoposide combination may be suitable for treating gastric carcinoma in elderly patients and patients whose comorbidity rates limit the application of other cytostatic agents. In addition, the following experimental data would seem to justify the LV/5-FU/etoposide combination:

1. The synergistic effect of 5-FU and etoposide in vitro and in vivo,[20,21] and
2. No cross-resistance between 5-FU and etoposide in tumor models.[20]

The LV/5-FU/etoposide combination dosage suitable for phase II studies was ascertained, and initial data about the effectiveness of and tolerance to the latter combination gathered during a pilot study, which took into account the clinical and experimental data (Wilke, Preusser, Achterrath, et al, unpublished).

Patients and Methods

The results obtained from the pilot study indicate that the combination was safe and effective for elderly patients when administered according to the following dosage/application schedule:

LV	300 mg/m², IV, days 1–3
Etoposide	120 mg/m², IV, days 1–3
5-FU	500 mg/m², IV, days 1–3

Therapy interval: Days 22–28 depending on the recovery of leukocytes and thrombocytes.

A total of 22 patients with advanced gastric carcinoma have been treated to date with the combination following the above dosage/application schedule during the subsequent disease-oriented phase II study. In addition to elderly patients (older than 65 years) younger patients who could not be treated with anthracyclines due to comcomitant cardiac disease were included in the study as well. Patient characteristics are outlined in Table 4. Response to therapy (remission, duration of remission) and side effects were evaluated according to WHO criteria.[22]

Endoscopy, CT, and ultrasound were employed to measure tumor localization. Scintigraphically suspect bone areas were checked via x-rays. Measurable tumor parameters were checked prior to admission into the study, before every therapy cycle, 4 weeks after the last course of therapy, and thereafter in 3-month intervals using the same methods employed during the initial examination. The hematologic parameters, kidney, liver, and heart function as well as plasma electrolytes were checked prior to the initiation of therapy, before each therapeutic cycle, and 4 weeks after the termination of therapy. Hematologic parameters (CBC, thrombocytes) were checked weekly. All patients who completed one therapeutic cycle were included in the evaluation of side effects in case of progressive disease. The administration of two courses of therapy was the precondition for evaluating the effectiveness of chemotherapy in all remaining patients. Side effects could be analyzed in all 22 patients and tumor response in 21.

Table 4. Patient characteristics

Age	Mean age 67 years (range 48–75)
> 65 years of age	15
≤ 65 years of age	7
Sex (male:female)	14:8
Karnofsky	Mean 70% (range 60–100%)
Local advanced inoperable primary tumor	5
Inoperable and distant metastases	17

Table 5. Therapy results with LV/5-FU/etoposide combination (n = 21)

CR	3 (14%)
CR + PR	9 (43%)
MR + NC	6 (29%)
PD	6 (29%)
CR + PR:	
Local advanced inoperable primary tumor	3/5 (60%)
Inoperable and distant metastases	6/16 (38%)
Remission by age:	
> 65 years	6/14 (43%)
≤ 65 years + heart disease	3/7 (43%)

MR = minor remission.
NC = no change.
PD = progressive disease.

Results

A total of 79 therapy cycles (average 3.5 per patient) were administered (Table 5). Three (14%) complete remissions and six (29%) partial remissions were achieved in 21 evaluable patients, yielding an overall remission rate of 43% (95% confidence limit, 23–63%). A minor response or arrest of growth was achieved in six other patients. Median duration of remission was 8 months and median survival time for all patients 9.5 months. Patients who responded with remission or arrest of growth lived a median of 10.5 months, while those with progressive disease survived a median of 4 months.

The side effects observed in the 22 evaluable patients are presented in Table 6. The LV/5-FU/etoposide combination therapy was well tolerated. No life-threatening WHO grade 4 side effects were observed. WHO grade 3 leukocytopenia and thrombocytopenia occurred in three and one patients, respectively. WHO grade 3 diarrhea was observed in two patients, while 12 (54%) experienced WHO grade 3 alopecia. Nausea/vomiting and mucositis (WHO grades 1 and 2) occurred in 55% and 28% of the patients, respectively. No cardiovascular, renal, pulmonary, hepatic, or CNS side effects were observed.

Table 6. Side effects of the LV/5-FU/etoposide combination (WHO grades), n = 22

	WHO grade			
	1	2	3	4
Alopecia	2 (9%)	7 (32%)	12 (54%)	0
Nausea/vomiting	7 (32%)	5 (23%)	0	0
Mucositis/stomatitis	3 (14%)	3 (14%)	0	0
Diarrhea	2 (9%)	1 (5%)	2 (9%)	0
Leukocytes	5 (23%)	8 (36%)	3 (14%)	0
Thrombocytes	5 (23%)	2 (9%)	1 (5%)	0

Discussion

Polychemotherapy with the FAM, FAMe, FAMTX, FAP, FAB, and EAP protocols, the most frequently employed against gastric carcinoma (see Table 2), should be limited to selected patients in controlled trial conditions because of their constituent side effects and tolerance only in selected patient populations. Elderly patients (older than 65 years of age) and patients with impaired organ function (heart, kidneys, liver, lungs) are often excluded from treatment with aggressive chemotherapy programs to avoid serious side effects.

Approximately 60% of patients with gastric carcinoma are older than 65 years of age and suffer from one or more age-related tumor-independent organ diseases, primarily caused by impaired functioning of the cardiovascular, renal, hepatic, and respiratory systems. These data suggest that only 20% to 30% of all gastric carcinoma patients can be treated with the polychemotherapy protocols commonly in use today. Development of an effective chemotherapy with acceptable side effects for the majority of patients is therefore a pressing therapeutic problem.

After analyzing the side effects exerted by cytostatic drugs active against gastric carcinoma, the LV/5-FU/etoposide combination was developed and tested in an ongoing phase II study of the treatment of elderly patients and those with concomitant cardiac disease.

A remission rate of 43% (including 14% complete remissions) was achieved in 21 evaluable patients. Median duration of remission was 8 months, and median survival time for all patients 9.5 months. Life-threatening hematologic side effects and/or serious nonhematologic organ toxicity as well as irreversible side effects were not observed.

The LV/5-FU/etoposide combination appears to be suited for the treatment of specific high-risk patients who cannot be treated with the usual combinations. Preliminary results suggest that remission rates and median survival times similar to those attained with FAM, FAMe, FAP, FAB, and FAMTX may be achieved with the LV/5-FU/etoposide combination in specific high-risk patients under study conditions.

These initial experiences with the LV/5-FU/etoposide combination indicate that relatively well-tolerated chemotherapy programs for elderly patients and younger patients with specific organ diseases not caused by tumors may be developed by careful selection of currently available cytostatic drugs.

The attempt to develop a risk-related strategy from the standpoint of differential therapy in cases of gastric carcinoma should be carried over to the treatment of other malignant growths, since only about 20% of all patients with malignant tumors may be treated by means of aggressive polychemotherapy within studies.

The development of such chemotherapy programs should focus on cytostatic agents having a high therapeutic index and nonoverlapping side effects.

References

1. Statistisches Bundesamt Wiesbaden: Gesundheitswesen, Fachserie 12 Todesursachen 1983. Statistisches Bundesamt. Wiesbaden, W. Kohlhammer, Stuttgart, 1984, p 12.
2. Waterhouse JAH: Epidemiology of gastric cancer, in Preece PE, Cuschieri A, Wellwood JM (eds): Cancer of the Stomach. London, Grune & Stratton, 1985, p 1.
3. Hunter CP, Frelick RW, Feldman AR, et al: Selection factors in clinical trials: results from the community clinical oncology program physician's patient log. Cancer Treat Rep 1987;71:559.
4. Lee YJ, Catane R, Rozencweig M, et al: Analysis and interpretation of response rates for anticancer drugs. Cancer Treat Rep 1970;63:1713.
5. Walder S, Green M, Muggia F: The role of anthracyclines in the treatment of gastric cancer. Cancer Treat Rev 1985;12:105.
6. Queisser W, Flechtner H: Chemotherapy of advanced gastric carcinoma. Onkologie 1986;9:319.
7. DeSimone PA, Gams R, Birch R: Phase II evaluation of mitoxantrone in advanced carcinoma of the stomach: a Southwestern Cancer Study Group trial. Cancer Treat Rep 1986;70:1043.
8. Louie AC, Issell BF: Amsacrine (AMSA) – a clinical review. J Clin Oncol 1985;3:562.
9. Aisner J, Van Echo DA, Whitacre J, et al: A phase I trial of continuous infusion VP16-213 (Etoposide). Cancer Chemother Pharmacol 1982;7:157.
10. Greco FA, Johnson DH, Hande RK, et al: High-dose etoposide (VP-16) in small-cell lung cancer. Sem Oncol 1985;12(suppl 2):42.
11. Kelsen DP, Magill G, Cheng E, et al: Phase II trial of etoposide (VP16) in the treatment of upper gastrointestinal malignancies, abstract. Proc ASCO 1982;96:C-371.
12. Seeber S, Osieka R, Schmidt CG, et al: In vivo resistance towards anthracyclines, etoposide, and cis-diaminedichloroplatinum (II). Cancer Res 1982;67:4719.
13. Tozak LK, Von Hoff DD: The cardiotoxicity of anticancer agents, in Perry MC, Yabro JW (eds): Toxicity of Chemotherapy. Orlando, Grune & Stratton, 1984, p 199.
14. Franke H: Wesen und Bedeutung der Polypathie und Multimorbidität in der Alterscheilkunde. Internist 1984;25:451.
15. Lipschitz DA: Conference: cancer in the elderly: basic science and clinical aspects. Ann Intern Med 1985;102:218.
16. Vestal RE: Drug use in the elderly: a review of problems and special considerations. Drugs 1978;16:358.
17. Gallmeier WM: Krebstherapie im Alter. Mun Med Wochens 1977;43:1379.
18. Douglass HO, Trave F, Milliron S, et al: A phase II trial of 5-fluorouracil and high-dose intravenous leukovorin in gastric carcinoma. J Clin Oncol 1987;5:1150.
19. Machover D, Goldschmidt E, Chollet P: Treatment of advanced colorectal and gastric adenocarcinomas with 5-fluorouracil and high-dose folinic acid. J Clin Oncol 1986;4:685.
20. Hill BT: Potential of continuous tumor cell lines for establishing patterns of cross-resistance and collateral sensitivity in vitro. Drugs Exp Clin Res 1986;12:293.
21. Osswald H, Kunz W: Therapeutic synergism of etoposide and fluorouracil combined sequentially in advanced leukemia L1210, abstract. Cancer Res Clin Oncol 1987; 113(suppl):53;39.
22. World Health Organization: Handbook for Reporting Results of Cancer Treatment. WHO Offset Publication No. 48. World Health Organization, 1979, p 1.

Part V
Summary

CHAPTER 16

Consequences and Practical Procedures During Gastric Carcinoma: Record of Results from a Consensus Conference

J. Hotz, H.-J. Meyer, and H.-J. Schmoll

Primary Diagnosis (Table 1)

Endoscopy

Endoscopy is the method of choice for detecting gastric carcinoma. The endoscopist should describe the location and extent of the tumor as accurately as possible. The biopsy specimens must be as numerous and large as possible for classifying the histological type (eg, according to Laurén), and the possible occurrence of mixed intestinal and diffuse types considered. Histologic classification might well determine surgical procedure (see article by H.-J. Meyer) and should therefore be performed as soon as possible prior to surgery. Actual histologic classification and tumor stage determination then ensue intra- and postoperatively (see article by P. Hermanek).

In the case of a prospective partial resection (eg, in deep-seated carcinoma of the antrum), biopsies should be taken from the proximal postoperatively remaining mucosa of the corpus to check for possible epithelial dysplasia. Early secondary gastric carcinoma must also be considered. Routine cytological brush smear is not necessary but makes sense in isolated cases in which the diagnosis of carcinoma is uncertain. Differential diagnosis of gastric lymphoma may occasionally be difficult, ie, in the case of an intensive lymphatic reaction to adenocarcinoma. An immunocytochemical examination with cytology must be carried out occasionally in these cases (P. Hermanek).

Preoperative Staging (Table 2)

Barium Meal

Radiology may provide important clues to possible wall infiltration in cases where scirrhous carcinoma is suspected, in particular with negative histology. This method need not be employed given a clear endoscopic identification of an adenocarcinoma in the middle and lower sections of the stomach. In high-seated carcinomas encompassing the cardia, preoperative radiologic examination of the upper gastrointestinal tract as well as endoscopy should be performed in each case.

Table 1. Primary diagnosis

Endoscopy-biopsy
Histological classification according to Laurén (intestinal type/diffuse type/mixed type) determines the margin of safety during resection
Positive biopsy of the remainder in the case of resection (cave secondary carcinoma in the residual stomach)
Cytology if diagnosis uncertain
Differential diagnosis of malignant lymphoma: Immunocytochemistry + cytology

Ultrasonic Examination of the Abdomen

This method is obligatory to clarify coarse regional lymph-node metastases, metastases in the liver, as well as possible ascites or Krukenberg's tumor in the ovary. Abdominal ultrasound is also helpful in evaluating depth of primary tumor infiltration into the wall. In no case can sonographic findings provide adequate information about resectability, inoperability, or precise clinical staging.

Computer Tomography

CT is unnecessary for routine preoperative diagnosis, since it determines neither the indication for surgery nor technique. Exceptions include evaluation of indication for surgery in at-risk patients and assessment of mediastinal lymphomas in the case of high-seated gastric carcinoma (thorax CT in addition! occasionally mediastinoscopy?). CT may additionally become necessary in the case of chemotherapy alone (see below) for precise staging prior to initiation of chemotherapy. (Reminder: Isolated liver metastases are very rare [2% to 5%] and cannot be resected successfully, as a result of which a combined sonographic and CT examination of the abdomen may be avoided.)

Laparoscopy

Laparoscopy makes sense only in exceptional cases when isolated liver metastases are suspected or for clarifying a peritoneal carcinosis.

Table 2. Necessary, possible, and unnecessary examinations for preoperative staging

Preoperative staging

- Barium meal in high-seated carcinoma
- Ultrasonography (lymph nodes, ascites, liver metastases?)
- No routine CT:
  Exception: High-seated tumor and risk patients
  (Isolated liver metastases very rare, CT therefore not obligatory.)
- No liver scan
- Bone scan only when clinical suspicion (eg, elevated AP)
- Tumor marker only for purposes of study

Liver Scan

Liver scanning is clearly inferior to ultrasonic examination of the abdomen or CT in terms of accuracy and is therefore obsolete.

Bone Scan

Bone scanning should not be performed routinely but only in clinically suspect cases (eg, ostealgia, elevated alkaline phosphatase given normal leucine-aminophosphatase, and gamma-glutamyl-transferase).

Determination of Tumor Markers (CEA, Ca 19-9)

Determination of tumor markers (CEA, Ca 19-9) is not necessary preoperatively and should be recommended only for the purposes of study, since the result influences neither the therapeutic procedure nor additional diagnostic measures. In contrast, postoperative evaluation of the result does make sense and is included in many postoperative care programs. (Reminder: Preoperative staging should be performed sparingly, since operations are as a rule primary ones. It may also become necessary to expand the staging process after surgery [ie, prior to deciding on additional chemotherapy]).

Surgical Treatment (Table 3)

Resectability should be evaluated intraoperatively in every case if possible, following the principle of removing as much tumor tissue as possible. Radicality of the surgery depends on tumor localization, extent, and histological type. In every case the goal should be gastrectomy in patients whose overall condition is good, particularly in those who are younger. The pathologist must be as careful as possible in analyzing the lymph-node material removed. (For further details we refer the reader to the chapters by H.-J. Meyer, J. Jähne, and R. Pichlmayr, by A. Hölscher, M. Schüler, and J.R. Siewert, and by G. Feifel and G. Schüder.)

Postoperative Care (Table 4)

A second operation for removing a mesenteric recurrence is technically impossible after a primary extensive resection on part of the stomach, particularly following gastrectomy. In contrast to the situation with carcinoma of the colon, for

Table 3. Recommended standard operations following diagnosis of gastric carcinoma

Resectability (TN?)
Radical surgery depending on localization, extent, histological type
Gastrectomy, given good condition

Table 4. Guidelines for postoperative follow-up after gastric surgery due to carcinoma

Individualized!
Sparing
Symptom-oriented
Prospective:
Close-meshed routine examinations prior to eventual chemotherapy

example, there are no additional possibilities for resecting isolated liver and lung metastases. This is because diffuse metastases are almost always present in patients with gastric carcinoma, even in those cases where the first solitary metastasis has been detected. Owing to the paucity of results for surgical treatment, given the detection of regional and organ metastases, postoperative care should be as symptom-oriented and as sparingly used as possible (see chapter by P. Schlag). This helps to avoid unnecessarily alarming the patient in the asymptomatic stage and cuts costs.

The postoperative care programs in common use throughout the Federal Republic of Germany should be reviewed with a critical eye with these facts in mind. A careful postoperative examination must be performed at regular intervals (ie, every 3 months or tightly symptom-oriented) if chemotherapy with a curative approach nonetheless becomes possible in the near future. In those cases where metastases have been detected and chemotherapy has been initiated, follow-up examinations must follow the standards of internal oncology. Advisable here is a combined sonographic-CT, radiologic (thorax), and scintigraphic bone examination which includes the determination of tumor markers (CEA, Ca 19-9).

Chemotherapy Procedures in Cases of Gastric Carcinoma (Table 5)

Standard Therapy

Standard therapy may not yet be recommended at the current level of knowledge. Reflecting only very low response rates, previous results obtained using the FAM protocol are indicated within the framework of a purely palliative treatment for alleviating symptoms. Treatment should be discontinued if the therapy is unsuccessful, especially when symptoms have not been alleviated (ie, despite quantifiable tumor regression) (see chapters by H. Wilke et al, P. Preusser et al).

Therapeutic Procedures with a Positive Outlook

The latest therapeutic results, particularly with the FAMTX and EAP protocols, indicate that it may be possible to employ intensified chemotherapy against

Table 5. Chemotherapeutic possibilities during gastric carcinoma

Standard therapy not yet established
New protocols with a positive trend
Resection + adjuvant chemotherapy
Resection + palliative (curative?) chemotherapy
Bulky disease: Chemotherapy + second look operation
Palliative (symptomatic) therapy in elderly inoperable patients

See text for details.

gastric carcinoma in the form of a tumor-sensitive chemotherapy. The results obtained from studies currently underway must be evaluated before any general recommendation can be made, however. Having already been shown to be superior, the experiences gained with the more recent protocols cited are making it possible to try both models "ex juvantibus" in patients whose overall condition is good with respect to their relatively good tolerance, especially in the case of the

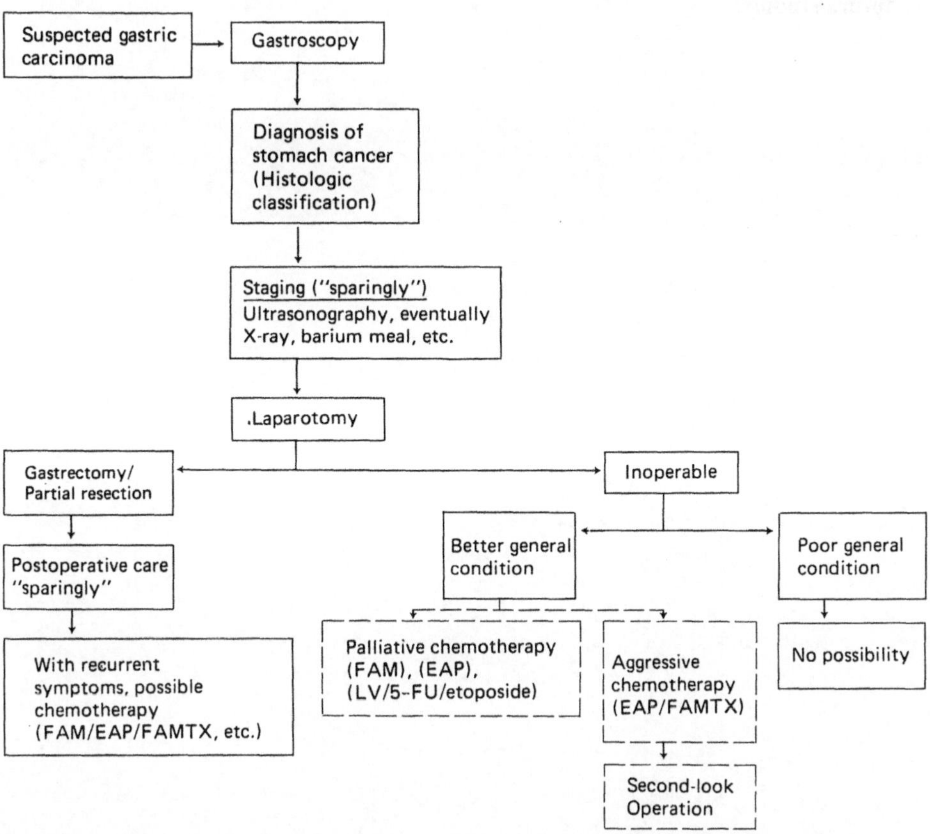

Fig. 1. Flow chart of procedure for patients with gastric carcinoma. See text for details.

EAP protocol. If the response is favorable after one or two courses, at least two and preferably four additional courses should follow. In patients older than 65 years whose overall condition is good, the protocol with leukovorin/5-FU/etoposide indicated by Preusser et al in this book can be recommended palliatively in cases of inoperability or following resections and given remaining tumor masses or relapses. The symptoms and overall level of suffering as well as the urgent request of the patient should serve as diagnostic guidelines.

The latest experiences employing the combination of surgery and chemotherapy (see chapter by H. Wilke/H.-J. Meyer) have resulted in the following alternatives for prospective use in the future:

Gastrectomy/partial resection + adjuvant chemotherapy, Gastrectomy/resection + palliative (curative?) chemotherapy

Bulky disease: Chemotherapy following exploratory laparotomy + Second-look operation and gastrectomy given detected remission.

One must make sure in these cases that the timing of the second operation is made as early as possible. The procedures just cited are still experimental, so that their effectiveness has yet to be determined based on the results of current and future studies.

Index

GPSR Compliance

The European Union's (EU) General Product Safety Regulation (GPSR) is a set of rules that requires consumer products to be safe and our obligations to ensure this.

If you have any concerns about our products, you can contact us on ProductSafety@springernature.com

In case Publisher is established outside the EU, the EU authorized representative is:

Springer Nature Customer Service Center GmbH
Europaplatz 3
69115 Heidelberg, Germany

Batch number: 10712230

Printed by Printforce, the Netherlands